Raw Family Signature Dishes

Other books by Victoria Boutenko
12 Steps to Raw Food
Green for Life
Raw Family (with the Boutenko family)

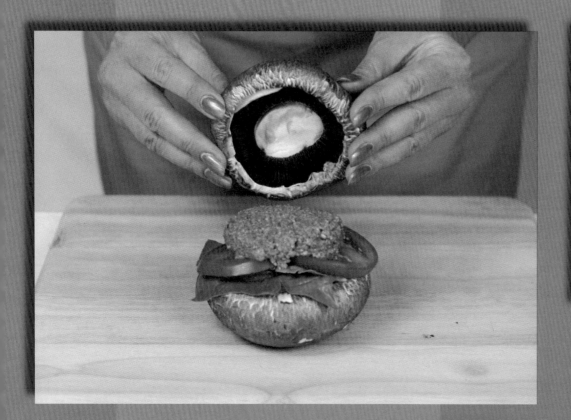
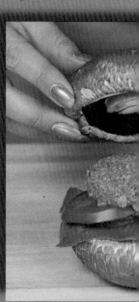

Raw Family Signature Dishes

A Step-by-Step Guide to Essential Live-Food Recipes

Victoria Boutenko

North Atlantic Books
Berkeley, California

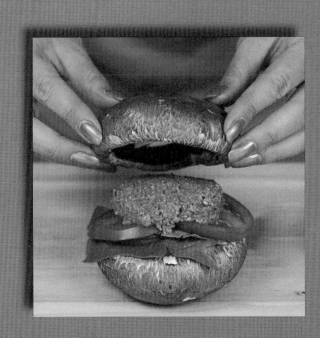

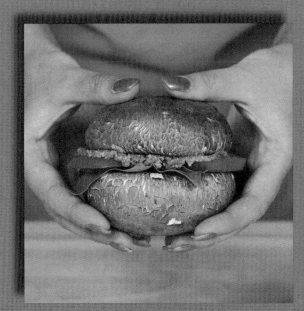

Published by
North Atlantic Books
P.O. Box 12327
Berkeley, California 94712

Cover and interior photos by Robert Petetit
Cover and book design by Linda Ronan
Printed in the United States of America

Raw Family Signature Dishes: A Step-by-Step Guide to Essential Live-Food Recipes is sponsored by the Society for the Study of Native Arts and Sciences, a nonprofit educational corporation whose goals are to develop an educational and cross-cultural perspective linking various scientific, social, and artistic fields; to nurture a holistic view of arts, sciences, humanities, and healing; and to publish and distribute literature on the relationship of mind, body, and nature.

North Atlantic Books' publications are available through most bookstores. For further information, visit our Web site at www.northatlanticbooks.com or call 800-733-3000.

Library of Congress Cataloging-in-Publication Data
Boutenko, Victoria.
 Raw family signature dishes : a step-by-step guide to essential live-food recipes / Victoria Boutenko.
   p. cm.
ISBN 978-1-55643-797-7
1. Raw food diet—Recipes. 2. Vegetarian cookery. I. Title.
RM237.5.B693 2009
641.5'63—dc22
               2008053430

1 2 3 4 5 6 7 8 9 United 14 13 12 11 10 09

*We dedicate this book to all those who
dare to explore new possibilities*

Contents

Foreword

For the last fifteen years Victoria Boutenko and her amazing "Raw Family" have been on a mission: to make live-food cuisine easy and accessible to as many people as possible. Traveling from city to city in their packed van, they have held countless seminars, classes, and chef trainings. Their events are notoriously affordable, yet at each one they feed people prodigious amounts of simple yet delicious food.

During this time, I have had the honor of sharing the kitchen at many gatherings with this remarkable "Raw Family," the Boutenkos. In every one of those kitchens, the presence of Victoria, Igor, Sergei, or Valya has made the food taste better—due not just to their immense live-food culinary skills, but also to the love and sincerity that they put into everything they do. Over the same period I have also witnessed Victoria somehow find time to publish groundbreaking book after book.

In *Raw Family Signature Dishes*, Victoria presents a selection of cornerstone recipes in the most comprehensive manner I have ever seen in a recipe book of any kind. Not only does Victoria lay out the equipment and ingredients needed to prepare each dish, but she also provides nutritional information and anecdotes about the recipe or key ingredients. Her introductions, which often take the form of an amusing or enlightening story, provide context for why each recipe forms part of a core set of live-food recipes for any aspiring raw chef's repertoire. The detailed step-by-step instruction clearly lays out each step with close-up color photos illuminating the process along the way. The result is a foolproof recipe book that will make live-food cuisine even more accessible to greater numbers of people around the world. While the recipes are precise, Victoria encourages readers to adapt her recipes to their own tastes and lifestyles, and offers variations for many of the recipes.

With *Raw Family Signature Dishes* Victoria has once again made a sincere offering of love for people and planet! She has taken her family's mission to the next level. *Raw Family Signature Dishes* makes time-tested healthy and delicious live-food absolutely simple and easy to make.

Bruce Horowitz
Author of *The Sun Kitchen Un-Cookbook*
www.thesunkitchen.com

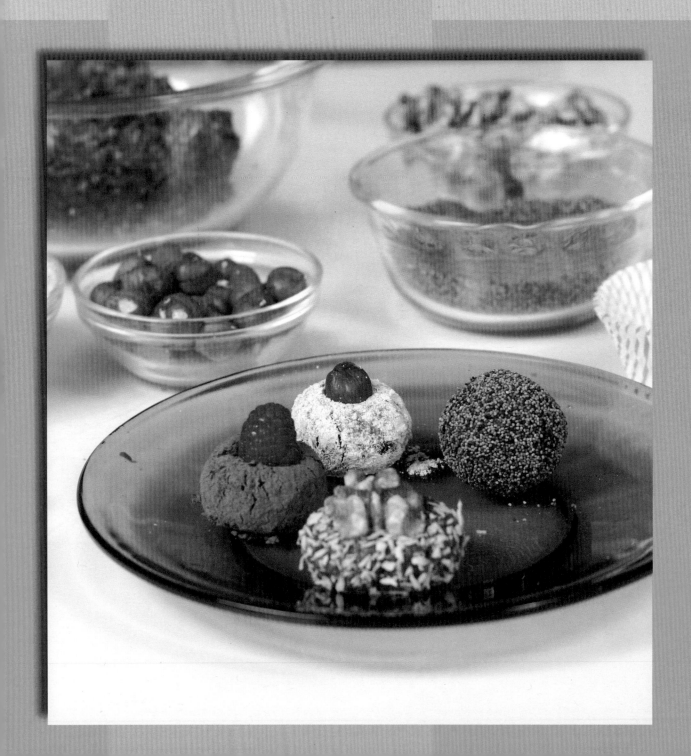

Introduction

Dear Reader,

I am excited to present this book to you. During fifteen years of living the raw food lifestyle my family and I have tried thousands of raw food recipes. The recipes we selected for this book were chosen because we consider them to be the core recipes for a raw food diet. Each has been retested and refined throughout the years.

We have published several raw food recipe books and conducted hundreds of food preparation demonstrations over the years. Many of our students have a strong desire to prepare raw food cuisine themselves and to introduce delicious raw meals to as many of their friends and family as possible. However, our readers have often told us that their own raw food dishes don't always turn out delicious even when they follow the recipes accurately.

So to make our recipes more accessible, we have illustrated these select dishes with photographs showing each step of preparation. It is our intention that any man, woman, or young adult, with or without cooking skills, will be able to prepare a tasty and nutritious raw meal and serve it in gourmet style.

We have included both simple and complex recipes here. While some of them are comparable to five-star restaurant servings, others are simple and practical. For example, we have included sprouting salad because this simple dish has served us many times in our lives, especially while traveling. Let me tell you a story that happened recently. We received an e-mail from an officer in the Middle East. He said that before he was deployed he had enjoyed a raw food diet, especially green smoothies. Now this young man found himself eating predominantly canned foods without any greens in sight. Our hearts went out to him. So we went to the local health-food store and purchased a small variety of sprouting seeds and mailed them with instructions to this young man. Within two weeks we received a raving letter from his entire troop that they had discovered a local source of sprouting seeds, which were now a staple of their diet.

My family and I invite you to try all of these dishes. Even though we provide you with exact instructions, we encourage you to experiment with the recipes and create your own variations.

In Health, Victoria Boutenko

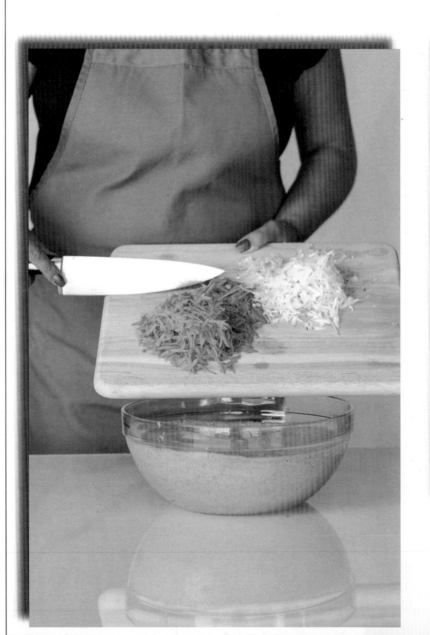
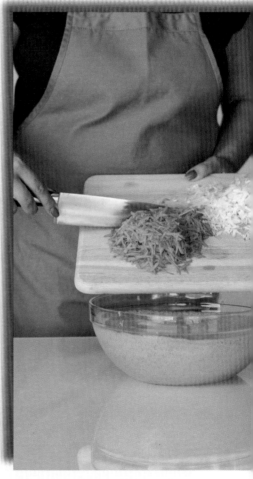

Recipes

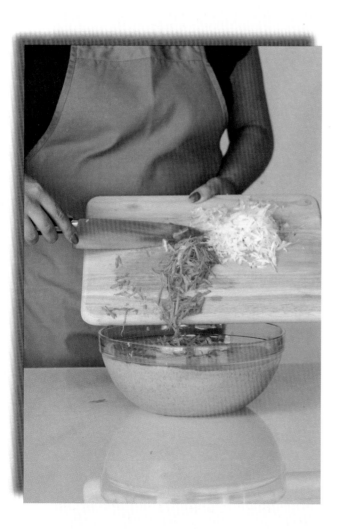

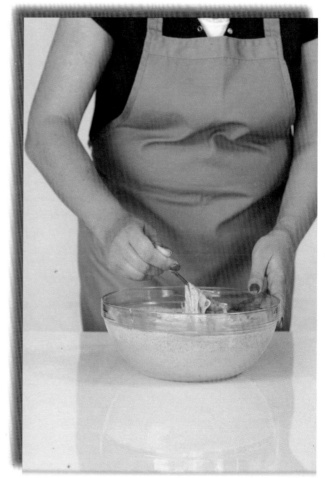

Salad History

Salt has been a traditional ingredient in salad dressings since ancient times. The very word "salad" derives from the Latin word for salt—*salata*. The earliest salads were wild greens and herbs seasoned with salt; these were the first vegetable foods available in spring and acted as a tonic after a dull winter diet. "Salted greens" came to mean "salad."

The ancient Greeks and Romans enjoyed a variety of dishes with raw greens and vegetables dressed with vinegar, oil, and herbs. In *Natural History*, for instance, Pliny the Elder reported that salads (*acetaria*) were composed of garden products that "needed no fire for cooking and saved fuel, and which were always ready" (*Natural History*, XIX, 58). They were easy to digest and designed to not overload the senses or stimulate the appetite.

The medical practitioners Hippocrates and Galen believed that raw vegetables easily slipped through the system and did not create obstructions for what followed, and so should be served as a first course.

Source: www.answers.com/topic/salad

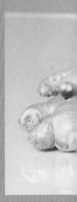

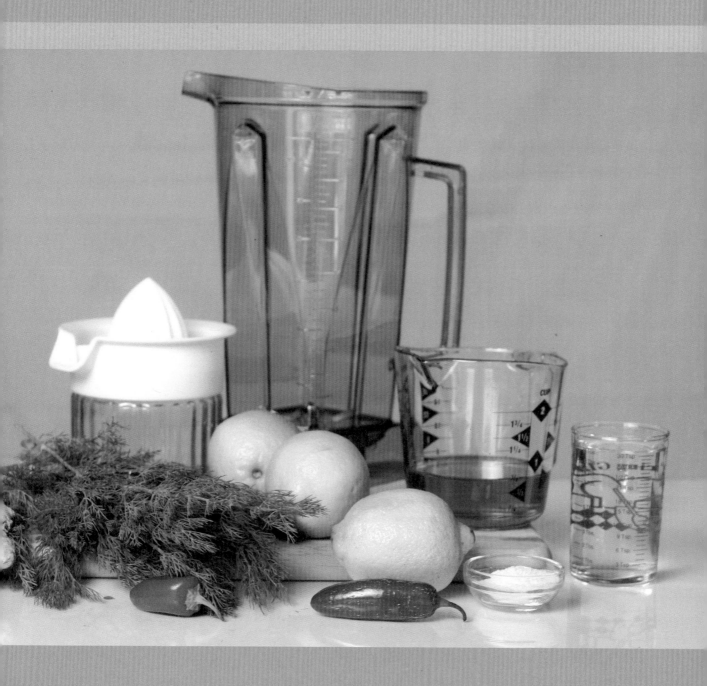

Salad Dressing and Simple Salad

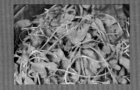
Dressing

The saying "dressing makes a salad" applies to raw salad dressing as well. The variety of flavors one can create in a raw food dressing is endless. Think of all the herbs, spices, and seasonings that exist in the world. Each one brings a different taste.

Raw salad dressing is one of the simplest recipes to make. It only takes a few minutes. To prepare a salad dressing, you will need:

Equipment

Blender
Lemon juicer
Bowl

Ingredients

½ cup lemon juice (about 2 lemons)
¼ cup olive oil
1 tbsp. raw agave nectar
1-inch piece ginger, unpeeled
1 or 2 hot peppers to taste (jalapeño or other)
1 bunch of parsley or dill
1 tsp. sea salt (optional)

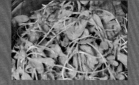

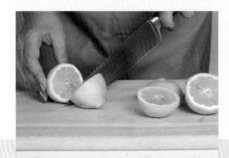

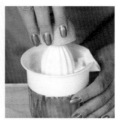

Slice the lemons in half and juice them.

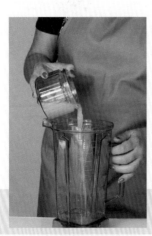

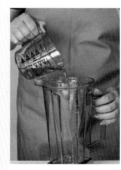

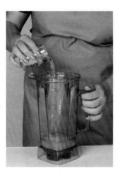

Pour the lemon juice, olive oil, and agave nectar into the blender.

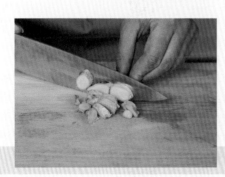

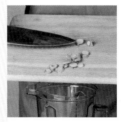

Chop ginger and add to the blender.

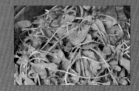
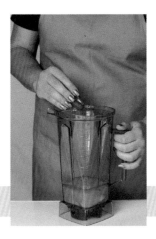

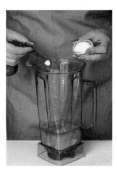

Destem the hot pepper and put it in the blender. Add sea salt.

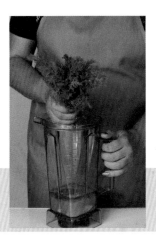

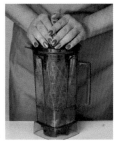

Add your parsley or dill to the blender. If you have a high-speed blender, you can put the entire bunch into the blender without chopping it.

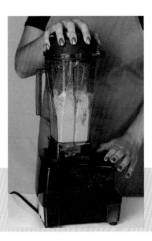

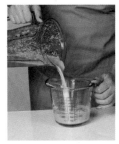

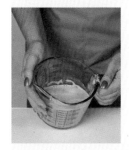

Secure the lid to the blender, and blend well. Pour the finished dressing into a jar. Makes about 1½ cups. Use immediately or keep refrigerated for up to one week.

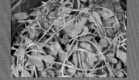

Simple Salad

Equipment
Cutting board
Knife
Bowl

Ingredients
1 bunch or head of any greens
Handful of any sprouts (sunflower, alfalfa, or other)
1 sunflower or other edible organic flower

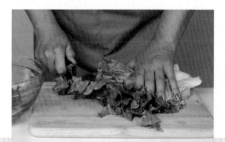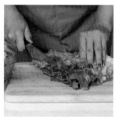

Chop (or tear) the greens into bite-size pieces and put them into the bowl.

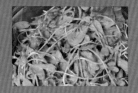

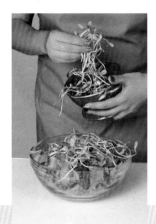
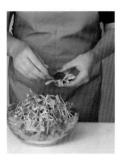

Add the sprouts and flower petals.

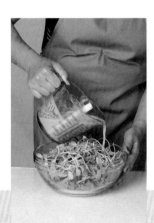
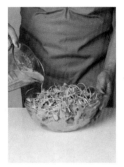

Pour the dressing evenly on the salad and toss. You may not need all of the dressing; add to taste. The salad should be eaten as soon as the dressing is added.

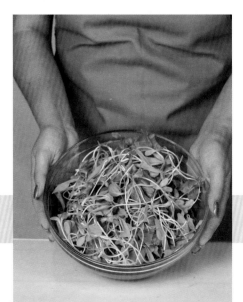

Without the dressing, the salad could be covered and kept in the refrigerator for one or two days.

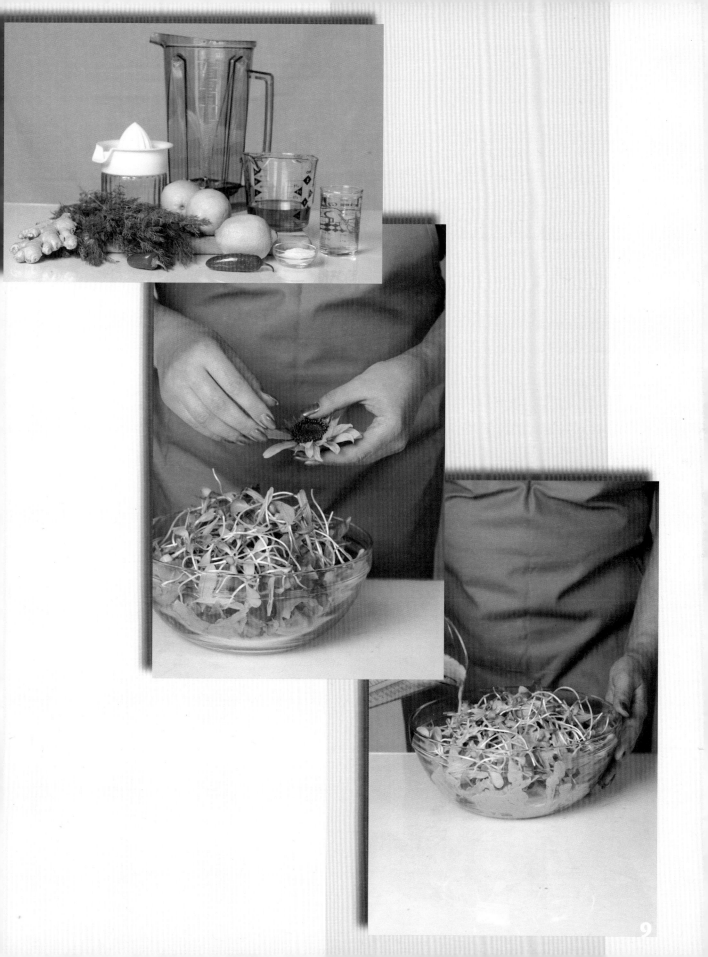

Nutritional Benefits of Sprouts

Sprouts possess a remarkable number of nutrients that are beneficial to human health.

According to the International Sprout Growers Association, Dr. Clive M. McKay, a nutrition professor at Cornell University, sparked interest in sprouts as a food source during World War II. He referred to sprouts as "a vegetable that will grow in any climate, will rival meat in nutritive value, will mature in three to five days, may be planted any day of the year, will require neither soil nor sunshine, will rival tomatoes in vitamin C, will be free of waste in preparation, and can be cooked with little fuel."

Together with a team of nutritionists, Dr. McKay dedicated many years of research to the amazing properties of sprouted soybeans. They found that sprouts retain the B-complex vitamins present in the original seed, and contain even more vitamin A than the seeds, and far more vitamin C than unsprouted seeds.

Source: www.isga-sprouts.org/index.html

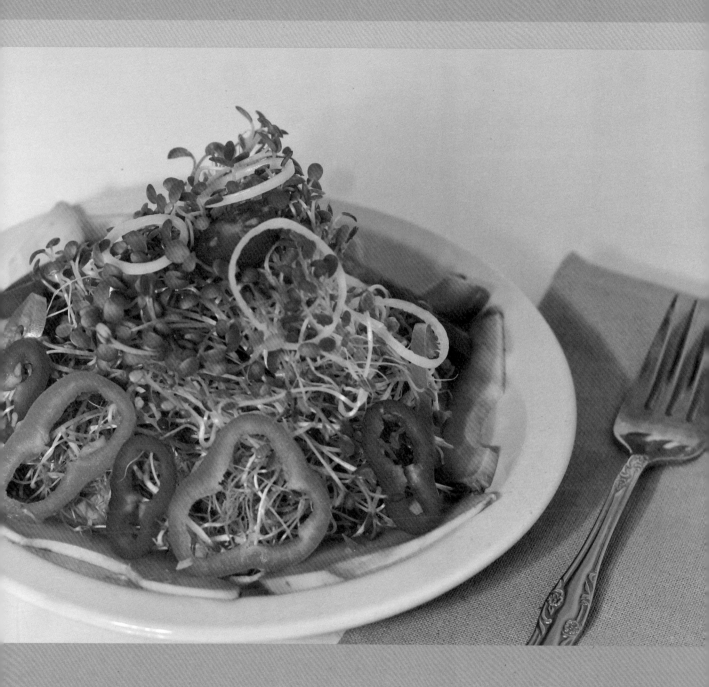

Sprouts and Sprouting Salad

Sprouts

Sprouts became one of the staples of our diet as soon as we tasted them and learned how easy they were to grow. In 1998, when we hiked the Pacific Crest Trail (2,650 miles), we had sprouts growing in our backpacks as we walked. We always have one kind of sprouts or another on our table.

Considering their cost and nutritional value, sprouts are the most economical food there is. For example, two tablespoons of alfalfa sprouts will grow into a quart of tightly packed greens, at the cost of about twenty cents. We prefer the simplest and least expensive way of sprouting: in glass jars. This recipe uses our family's favorite combination of sprouts, but many other variations are possible.

Equipment
3 1-quart glass jars
3 round pieces of mesh
    fabric or cheesecloth
3 rubber bands

Ingredients
2 tbsp. alfalfa sprouting seed
2 tbsp. fenugreek sprouting seed
2 tbsp. radish sprouting seed
Water as needed

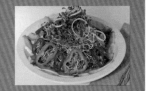
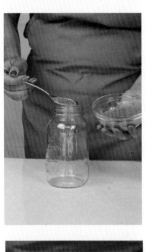
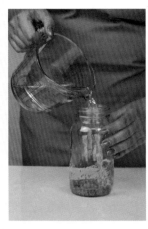
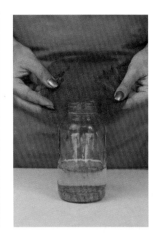
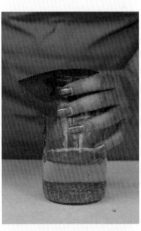
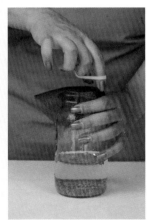
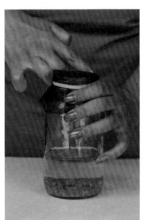
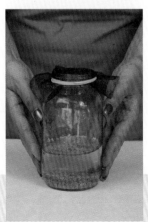
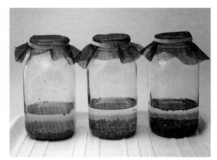

Day 1

Soak your seeds in approximately 2 cups of water per jar for about 12 hours. It is convenient to soak sprouting seeds in the evening. Cover the mouths of the jars with the mesh fabric and secure them with rubber bands. If you have very thin rubber bands, use 2 rubber bands on each jar. Keep your sprouting seeds away from direct sunlight.

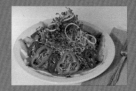

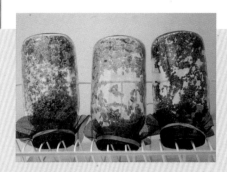

Day 2

Twice a day, in the morning and in the evening, pour the water out and rinse the seeds. To rinse your sprouting seeds, fill each jar with cool (or room temperature) water.

Gently tip the jar upside down several times. Pour water off and repeat once or twice.

Place the jars with seeds still inside on a dish rack at a 45-degree angle, bottom side up. This way the excess water can continue to drain while the air flows in freely.

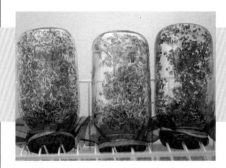

Day 3

Rinse sprouts twice a day with water. Drain the water and place the sprouts back at a 45-degree angle. You will see the sprouts growing quickly in mass.

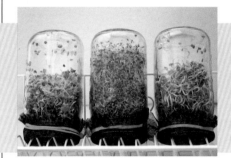

Day 4

Keep rinsing your sprouting seeds twice a day. When you notice some green leaves on your sprouts, move the jars to a brighter location for further greening, but not under a lot of direct sunlight. You will be amazed how little sunshine is needed to turn your sprouts green.

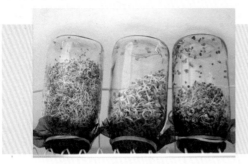

Day 5

The time to grow sprouts may vary between 3 to 6 days depending on the temperature in the room. The warmer the air is, the faster your sprouts will grow.

Keep rinsing your sprouting seeds twice a day until the tails grow twice the length of the seeds.

Enjoy delicious and nutritious sprouts in your salads. Place the extra sprouts in Tupperware or a Ziploc bag and keep them in the fridge for up to a week.

You may toss your sprouts with a little oil and vinegar or your favorite dressing. Try rolling sprouts together with a variety of veggies into collard leaves or nori sheets.

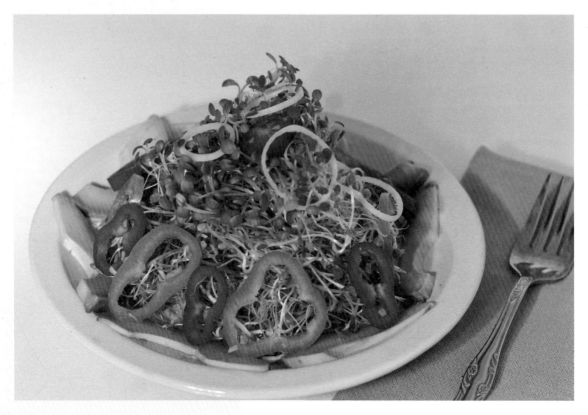

The Benefits of Flaxseed

In making raw bread, many chefs prefer to use flaxseed over grains or other seeds. Flaxseed is a perfect addition to the human diet because of its multiple health benefits.

According to the USDA, flaxseed is high in protein. One cup of flaxseed satisfies 92 percent of human adult needs in all essential amino acids, comparable to meat. Flaxseed is one of the best sources of essential fatty acids (Omega-3 and Omega-6). Furthermore, flaxseed contains an abundance of manganese, magnesium, phosphorus, selenium, zinc, iron, calcium, and other invaluable minerals. Flaxseed provides high amounts of B vitamins, particularly thiamine, all of which are essential for the health of the nervous system. Flaxseed is also nature's richest source of plant lignan, an important anticancer phytonutrient.

Flaxseed is very high in both soluble and insoluble fiber. The U.S. recommended daily allowance for fiber is thirty grams per day. Twenty-six percent of flaxseed is fiber. Just one-eighth of a cup of flaxseed contains six grams of fiber. Much research on dietary fiber has been done all around the world since the beginning of the twentieth century. We now have undeniable evidence of fiber's many healing properties. Here are some of them:

- Fiber can strengthen a diseased heart
- Fiber reduces cholesterol, which decreases the risk of heart disease
- Fiber prevents many different kinds of cancer and binds carcinogens
- Fiber can lessen the risk of diabetes and improve already diagnosed diabetes
- Fiber steadies blood-sugar levels by slowing down the absorption of sugar
- Fiber can strengthen the immune system
- Fiber keeps our bowels healthy, relieves constipation, and promotes regularity
- Fiber promotes healthy intestinal bacteria
- Fiber helps us lose weight and curbs overeating

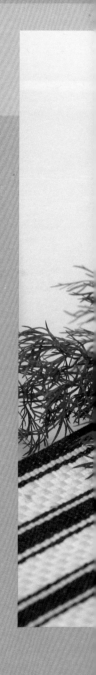

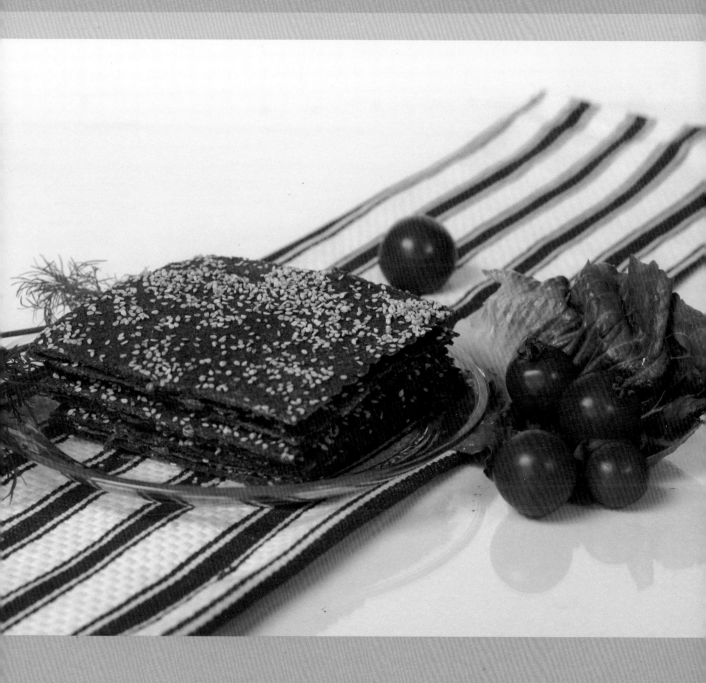

Igor's Live Flat Bread

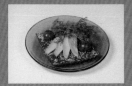
Igor's Live Flat Bread

OUR FAVORITE CRACKERS

Our family has been adding flaxseed to our meals every day either in the form of crackers or as flax meal. We have created a method of making flax crackers that taste like pumpernickel, our favorite Russian caraway bread.

In this chapter we share with you Igor's best cracker recipe, perfected over the years. Making a tasty raw cracker can often be tricky and challenging. If you follow this detailed guide closely, you should end up with good-tasting bread. As Igor likes to say, learn to make these delicious crackers and you will never be lonely!

Please note: in this text we will refer to Igor's live bread both as crackers and as bread. The only difference between the two is that the cracker is a drier, crunchier form of bread.

Equipment

Dehydrator
Blender
Coffee grinder (for grinding flaxseed if you don't have a high-speed blender)
Citrus juicer
Large bowl
Medium bowl for soaking raisins
2½-cup measuring container
Wooden spoon
Spatula
Cutting board
Large paring knife
Butter knife
Chopstick

Ingredients

7 cups water
2 pounds carrots (4–5 carrots)
1 bunch celery
1 head of garlic (8 large cloves)
1 large onion
½ cup lemon juice
2 jalapeño peppers
2 tbsp. sea salt (optional)
1 ½ cups raisins
7 cups flaxseeds
1 tbsp. caraway seeds
1 tbsp. coriander seeds
1 cup sesame seeds, hulled or unhulled

Yields: 81 pieces of 4.5 x 4.5–inch bread/cracker, which equals enough dough to fill a nine-tray Excalibur dehydrator.

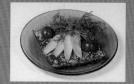

Preparing the Dough

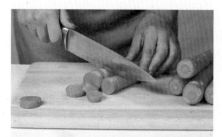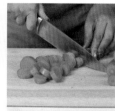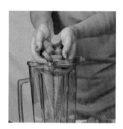

Slice the carrots into approximately ¼-inch slices. Carrots are a key ingredient in many dried cracker recipes. They make the crackers pliable and fluffy. Place the carrot slices in a blender. It should be about halfway full.

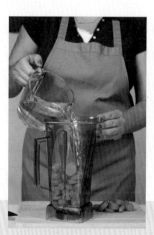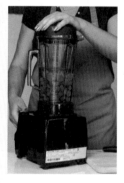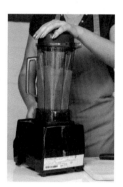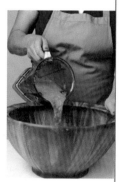

Cover the carrot pieces with water, approximately 3 cups. Blend the carrots until they become a thick, smooth liquid. Pour this mixture into a large bowl.

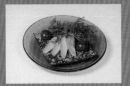

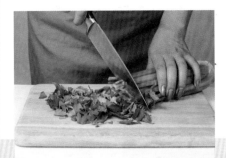
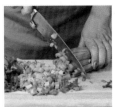
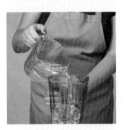

Cut 1 bunch of celery into approximately ½-inch pieces. We recommend cutting the celery into smaller pieces in order to use less water when blending.

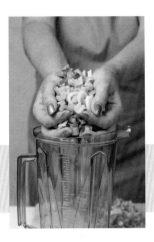
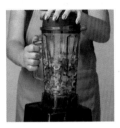
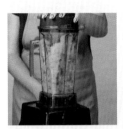
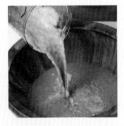

Add the pieces to the blender, cover them with water (approximately 2 ½ cups), and blend until smooth. Pour the celery mixture into the same bowl as the carrots.

We use celery because it is the finest source of nourishing organic sodium available in nature. Most people are lacking in organic sodium, which cannot be obtained from table salt because the body cannot properly assimilate sodium in this form.

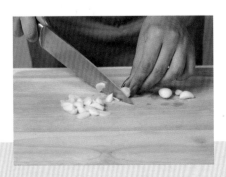
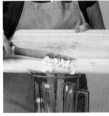

Peel 8 or 9 large cloves of garlic. Chop them into pieces and place them in the blender.

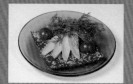

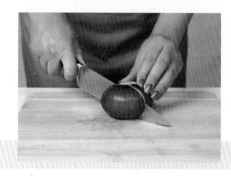
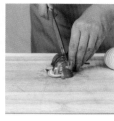
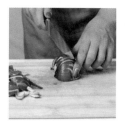

Peel 1 large onion and slice it into rough-chop pieces.

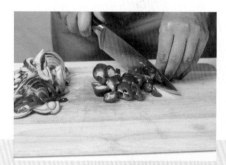
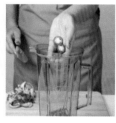
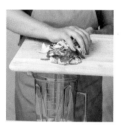

Cut up 2 jalapeño peppers (with seeds) and place them in the blender along with the onions and 2 tablespoons of sea salt.

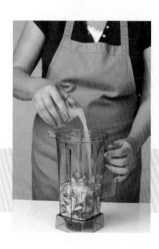
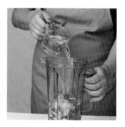

Juice 2 large lemons and add the juice to the blender. Add enough water to fully submerge the garlic and onion pieces.

This may seem like a lot of garlic and onion, but in the process of dehydration the strong garlic/onion smell and spiciness disappear. There will be hardly any of their taste left. If you prefer not to use garlic or onion, you may substitute them with another spicy ingredient such as jalapeño or ginger.

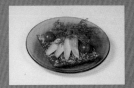
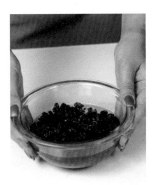
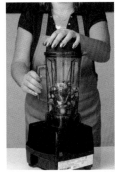
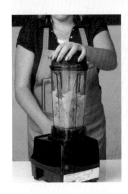
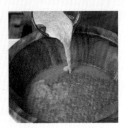

Soak 1½ cups of raisins in water for 20 minutes. Make sure they are completely submerged. In about 20 minutes the raisins will soften and the water will become light brown.

Blend the garlic, onion, and hot pepper and add to the mixture.

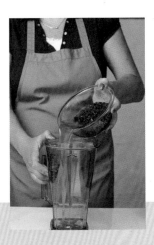
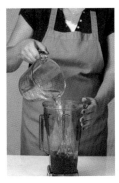
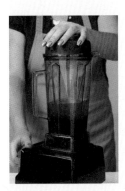

Pour the raisins and their soaking water into the blender. Add approximately 1½ cups of water to the blender. Raisins need a good deal of water to blend thoroughly.

You may use other sweeteners such as raw agave nectar or dates in these crackers. However, we prefer to use raisins because they add elasticity to the texture.

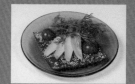

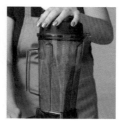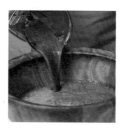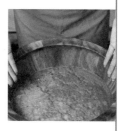

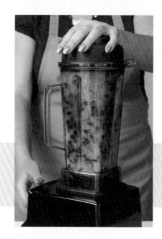

Blend the raisins till they are smooth, then pour them into the vegetable mix along with the blended carrots, celery, garlic, onion, and hot pepper. Set this veggie mix aside.

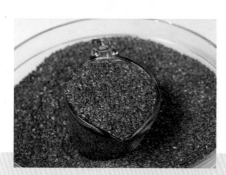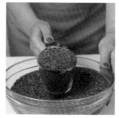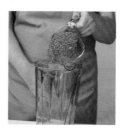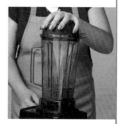

Grind up the seeds in your coffee grinder or high-speed blender. If you are grinding your flaxseeds in a high-speed blender, rinse out the container and wipe it dry with a paper towel or cloth. If you try to grind flaxseeds in a wet container, they will stick to the sides and refuse to grind up. Continue grinding the seeds 1 cup at a time until you have ground up all 7 cups. *Do not add water* to help the flaxseeds blend. It is important that they remain dry so they can absorb the water from the vegetable mix you have just made.

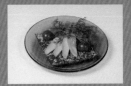
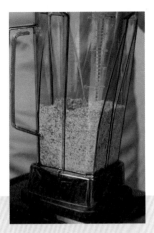

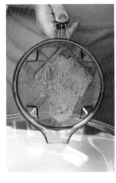

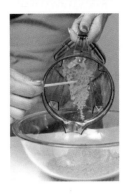

When emptying the blender, avoid touching the blades with any metal utensils. Contact with metal quickly dulls the blades. We have found that a wooden chopstick works best to get all of the ground flaxseed out.

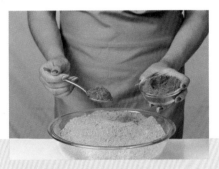

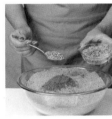

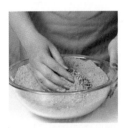

You now have 7 cups of flaxseed ground into fluffy, light-brown flour. To this, add 1 heaping tablespoon of ground caraway and 1 heaping tablespoon of coriander, mixing them in thoroughly.

Now prepare yourself for the trickiest and most critical part of making these crackers—mixing the dry and liquid parts together.

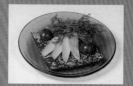

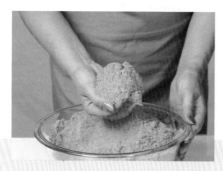 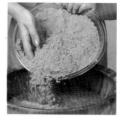 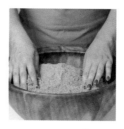

Pour the dry ground flaxseed into the bowl containing the blended veggies. Use your hands to quickly mix it all together. It is important to mix in the ground flaxseed last because if added first, it has a tendency to clump up into small globs that are difficult to get rid of. Clumpy crackers are still delicious, but they are not nearly as impressive-looking.

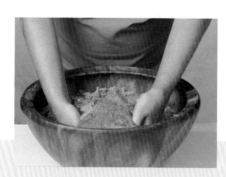 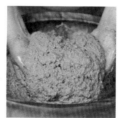

Continue mixing the dough until it becomes even in color and texture.

   At first the dough will not be very thick, but it will thicken within a few minutes as soon as the flaxseed gets a chance to absorb the juice from the vegetables.

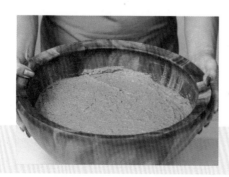

You don't want the dough to be too thick, because it will be difficult to spread onto trays.

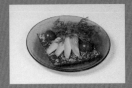

The Dehydrating Process

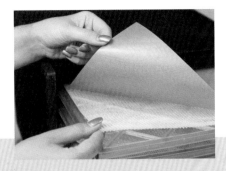

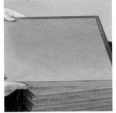

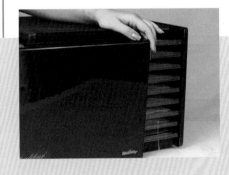

To prepare the dehydrator for drying crackers, take the trays out of your dehydrator and place a sheet of plastic mesh on each of them. Place a Teflex sheet or other nonstick sheet over the mesh.

Place a dehydrator tray with these two sheets (mesh and Teflex) on the counter.

We recommend using the nine-tray Excalibur dehydrator. A full batch of crackers in this dehydrator will last you at least two weeks. Using a smaller drying unit will force you to make smaller quantities of crackers more often. We have found the Excalibur to function better than any other dehydrator we have ever tried. The Excalibur dehydrator is light in weight, safe, uses a minimal amount of electricity, and dries food evenly. Excalibur dehydrators are easy to clean, if you know the trick—just soak the trays for twenty minutes in warm water and rinse off.

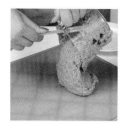

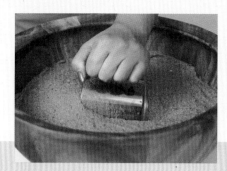 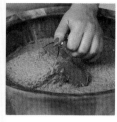 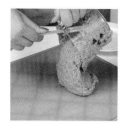

Using a 2½-cup measuring container to scoop up the cracker dough, pour the dough into the center of the tray. (Keep an extra plate handy for putting the empty measuring cup down when you don't need it to minimize the mess on your counter.)

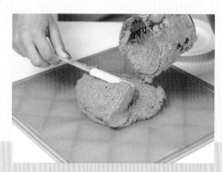 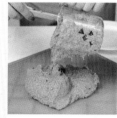 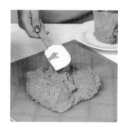 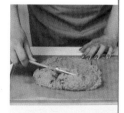

Use a spatula to spread the mixture from the center out towards the edges. A firm rubber spatula makes the job of spreading the cracker dough significantly easier. Spread the dough in an even layer ¼-inch thick. To spread the dough evenly, rotate the tray whenever you need to.

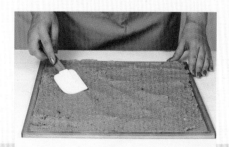 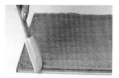 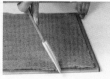 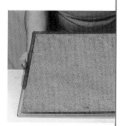

When all the dough is evenly spread, clean the edges of the tray with your spatula. This leaves less cleanup and makes it easier to remove the crackers from the tray when they are done.

27

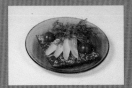
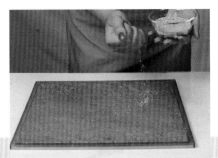
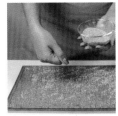
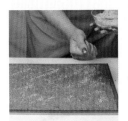
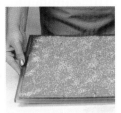

Your crackers will look a lot more appetizing if sprinkled with sesame seeds. You may use hulled or unhulled seeds. If you do not have access to sesame seeds, you may use pumpkin, sunflower, or flaxseed of a different color, such as golden flaxseed.

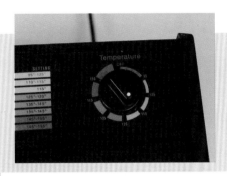

Set the temperature to 105 degrees F. Allow the crackers to dry for 10 to 12 hours. The speed of drying will vary depending on the temperature and humidity of your kitchen.

Keep checking on your crackers. When they are done, after approximately 10 to 12 hours of dehydrating, there should be darker, slightly moist (not sticky!) spots in the center of your cracker.

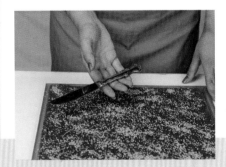
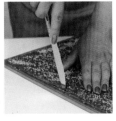

Remove the crackers from the dehydrator. To separate the cracker from the tray, you first need to cut the cracker edges loose. We have found that using a butter knife is the most effective way of doing this. Firmly press the butter knife down and slide it along the edge of the cracker.

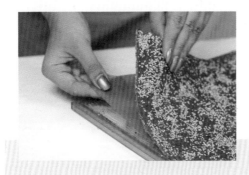
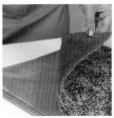

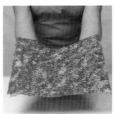

Once you have cut along all four edges of the cracker square, gently pull the cracker off the dehydrator tray. At this stage, the cracker is still soft enough to roll, as you can see in the picture.

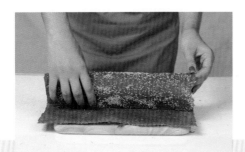

In our family we dehydrate our crackers to that magic consistency, when they are still flexible enough to be rolled. We call our crackers "bread" because that is what they taste and look like.

You may choose to dehydrate your cracker all the way to a crunchy consistency if you enjoy crunchy crackers better, especially if you are planning to travel. Fully dehydrated crackers will keep longer than moist ones. To thoroughly dehydrate the crackers to a crunchy texture, turn over the cracker and put it back on top of the mesh on the plastic tray without the Teflex layer. Place the crackers back in the dehydrator and continue drying them for another 2 to 4 hours.

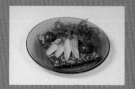

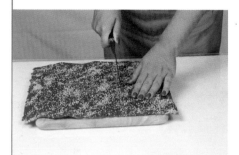

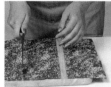

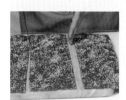

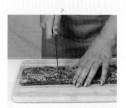

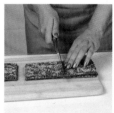

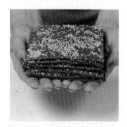

To cut the bread into equal pieces, place the cracker slab on a cutting board and use a serrated knife. We like to cut each of our bread slabs into nine pieces, as shown in these pictures. This method of cutting results in nine square (4.5 x 4.5–inch) crackers, a perfect size for making sandwiches.

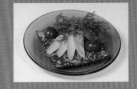

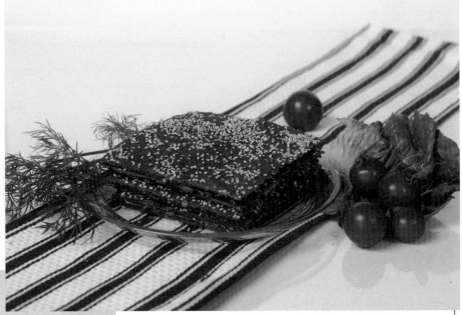

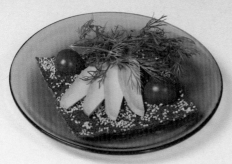

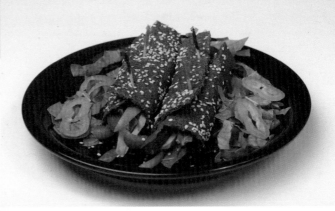

These pictures portray a few of the unlimited variations of serving tasty raw bread at your dinner table. Learning to make this bread will enable you to prepare various scrumptious healthy sandwiches or wraps in just minutes. Tasty live bread enriches any meal!

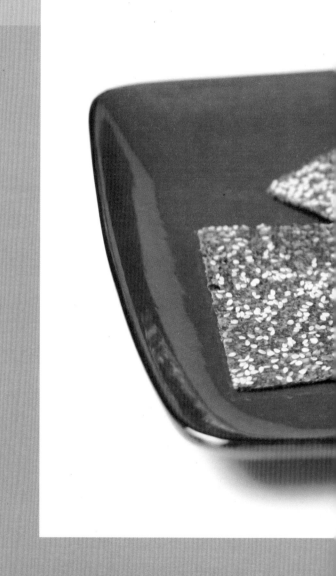

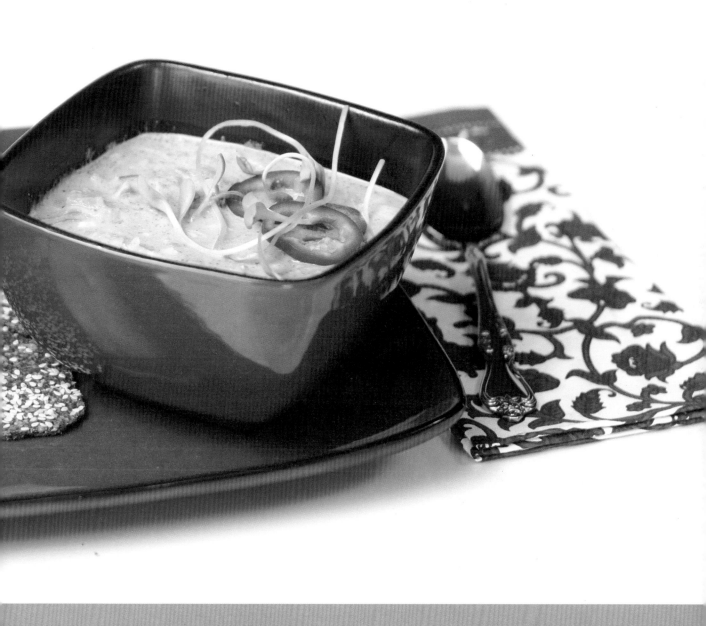

Soup

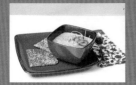
Soup

Similar to most cooked soups, raw soups are economical and easy to prepare. Raw soups are also exceptionally nutritious. There is a wide assortment of raw soup recipes created by an ever-growing number of raw chefs. Raw chilies, chowders, green soups, bisques, gazpachos, and stews have become popular daily choices for many health seekers.

We have chosen this particular recipe for its amazingly delicious taste. Everyone who has tried it enjoyed the bouquet of flavors and asked for a recipe. We hope you enjoy it too!

Equipment
Blender
Lemon juicer
Grater
Bowl
Cutting board
Knife

Ingredients

For stock:
3 cups water
¼ cup olive oil
4 medium-sized lemons
1 piece of fresh ginger, about 2 inches long
2 spicy peppers (jalapeño or other)
1 tsp. sea salt
8 Medjool dates
½ medium bunch celery
1 bunch cilantro

Remaining soup ingredients:
1 daikon radish
1 carrot
1 small turnip
1 piece (about 3 inches) of cauliflower
1 bell pepper (red, yellow, orange, or purple)
1 avocado

Ingredients for garnishing soup:
1 scallion
1 handful sprouts (sunflower, alfalfa, or other)
1 sweet pepper or 3 cherry tomatoes

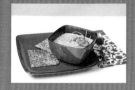

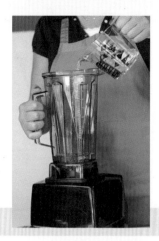 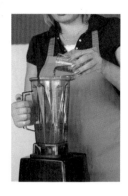

Pour water and olive oil into the blender.

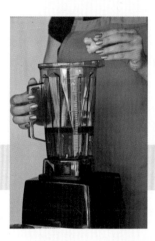 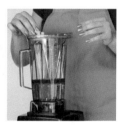

Place the ginger in your blender. The ginger does not need to be peeled if you have a powerful blender such as a Vita-Mix.

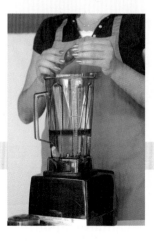 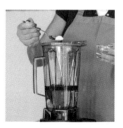

Add spicy peppers and sea salt to the blender.

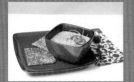
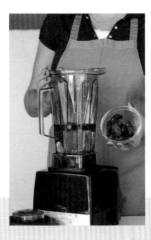
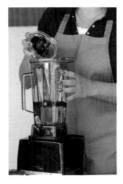

Remove the pits from the Medjool dates and add them to the blender. Be sure to take out the tails of the dates as well. They are rather woody and hard and don't blend well.

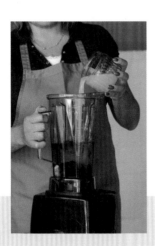

We prefer to use Medjools because of their delicate taste, but of course you may use any other kind of dates. If using smaller or less sweet dates, use 10 to 15.

Cut the lemons in half and juice them with a citrus juicer. This should make approximately 1 cup of lemon juice. Add the lemon juice to the blender.

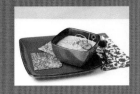
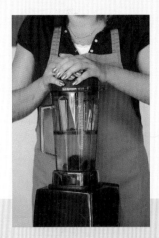 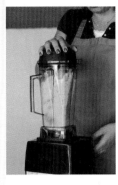

Secure the lid on the blender and blend all ingredients for 1 minute, or until smooth, on the highest speed of your blender.

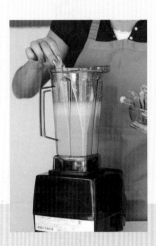 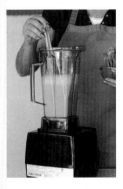 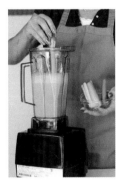 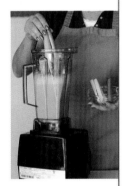

Place celery stalks in the blender, close the lid, and blend for about 20 to 30 seconds.

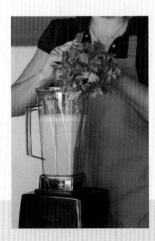 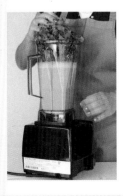

Place cilantro in the blender, close the lid, and blend for another 20 to 30 seconds.

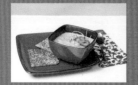
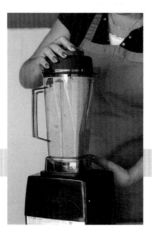

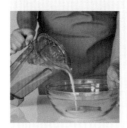

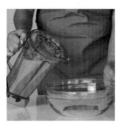

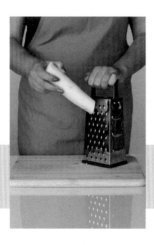

Now your stock is ready. Pour it into the bowl.

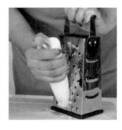

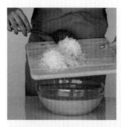

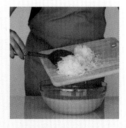

Grate the daikon. If you want your daikon to have long strands and look like noodles, make long strokes while grating it. Add your daikon "noodles" to the soup stock.

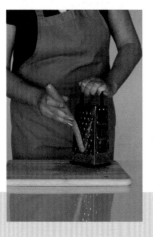

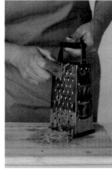

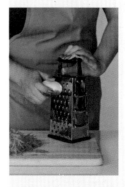

Grate the carrot and turnip. Grated carrots are a particularly important ingredient for almost any raw soup. They add a beautiful bright color and sweet taste and also make the soup look similar to a cooked soup.

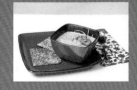

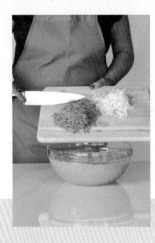
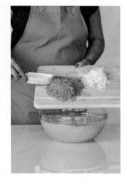
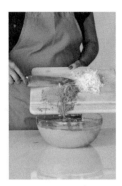
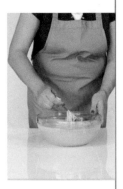

Add the carrot and turnip to the soup and stir, making sure that all grated veggies are completely submerged in the liquid so they don't oxidize and turn brown.

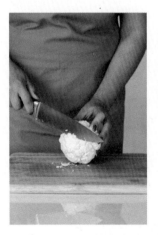
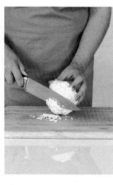
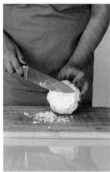
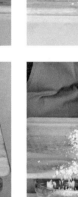

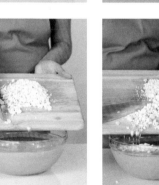

Thinly slice off the cauliflower florets and add them to the soup. Small cauliflower pieces add a nice crunchy texture.

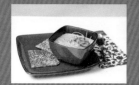
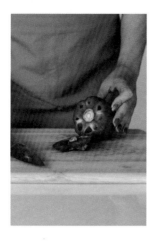 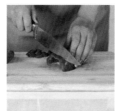 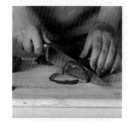 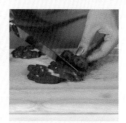

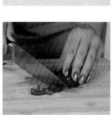 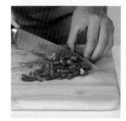 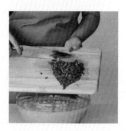

Remove stem and seeds from the bell pepper, dice into approximately ½-inch pieces, and add to the soup.

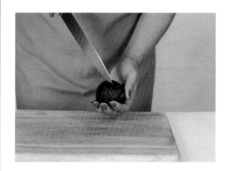 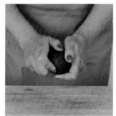 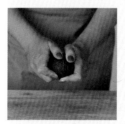 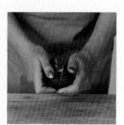

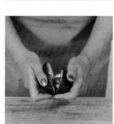

Cut the avocado in half. (A perfect avocado should not be too hard or too soft. It yields a little when lightly pressed with a finger.) Holding each side with a different hand, twist the avocado halves in different directions. This movement will divide the avocado into two equal parts, one with the seed and one without.

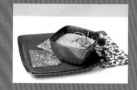

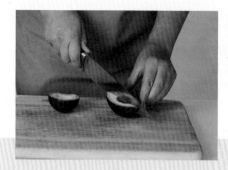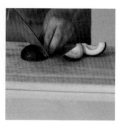

Hit the avocado seed lightly with the sharp side of your knife, so that the blade sticks in the seed. Twist the knife and the seed will easily come out of the avocado.

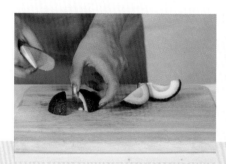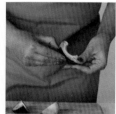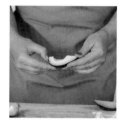

Cut each avocado half into quarters. At this point it should be easy to peel off the skin.

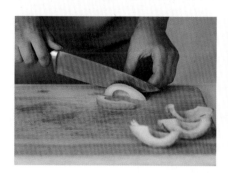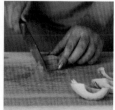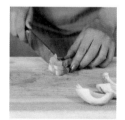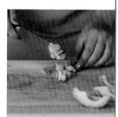

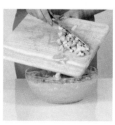

Cut the avocado into cubes and add to the soup. Some people say that avocado cubes in the raw soup resemble cooked potatoes in a traditional soup.

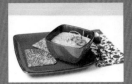

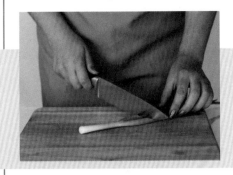

Now it is time to decorate your soup and make it look appealing to the eye. We recommend that you complete this last stage just before serving the soup, either in the large bowl or in individual serving bowls.

Thinly slice the scallions and sprinkle them across the surface of the soup.

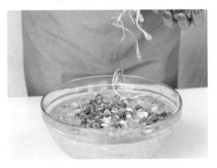 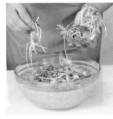 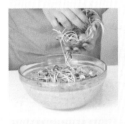 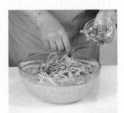

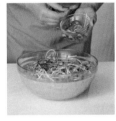 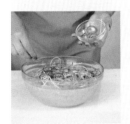

Place the sprouts evenly across the soup and arrange thinly sliced sweet peppers over the sprouts.

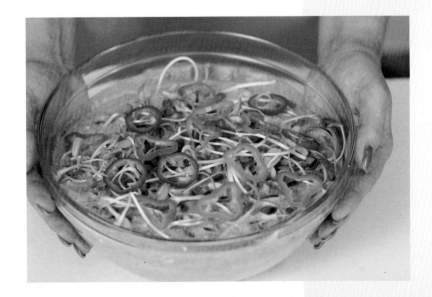

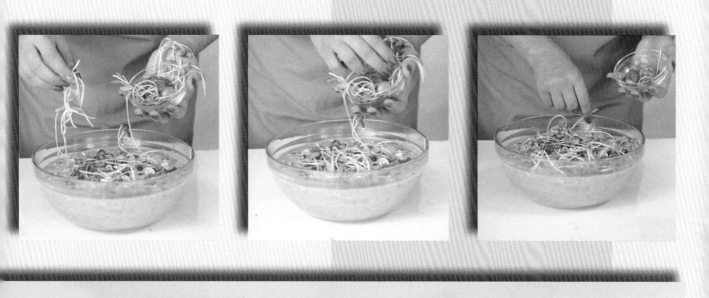

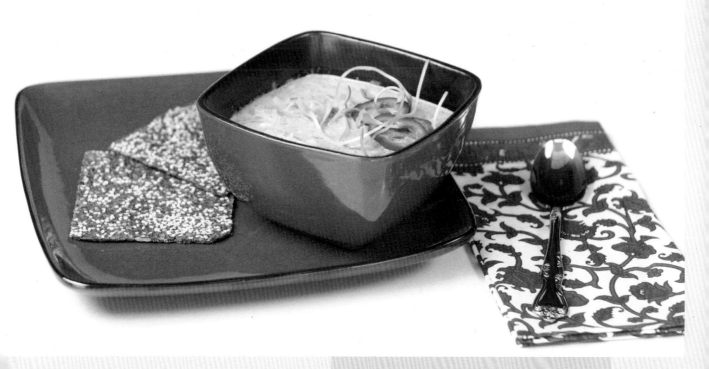

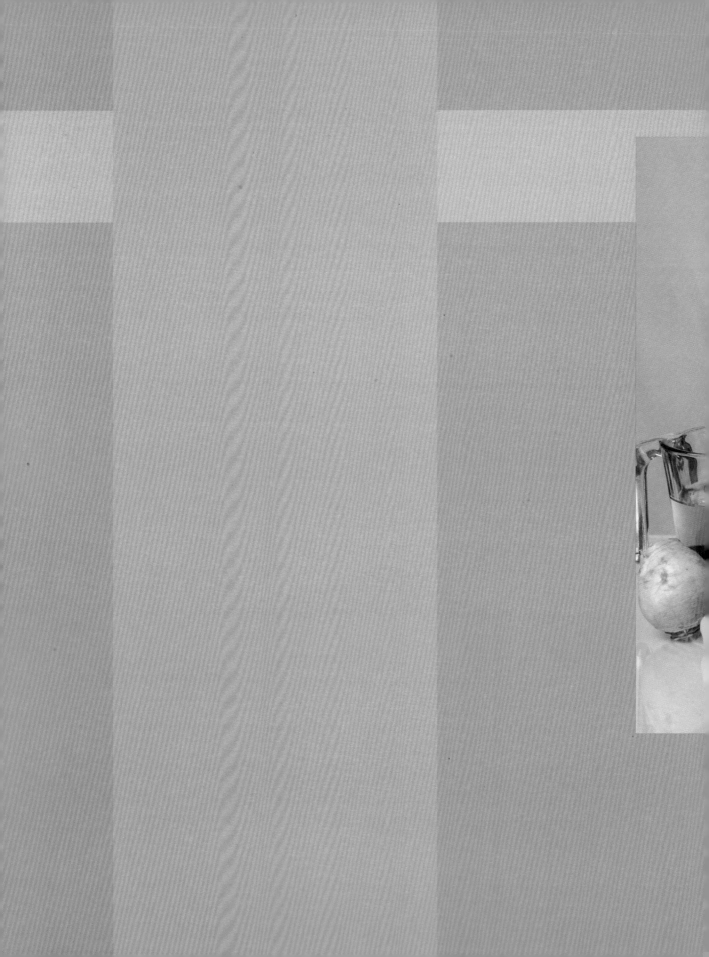

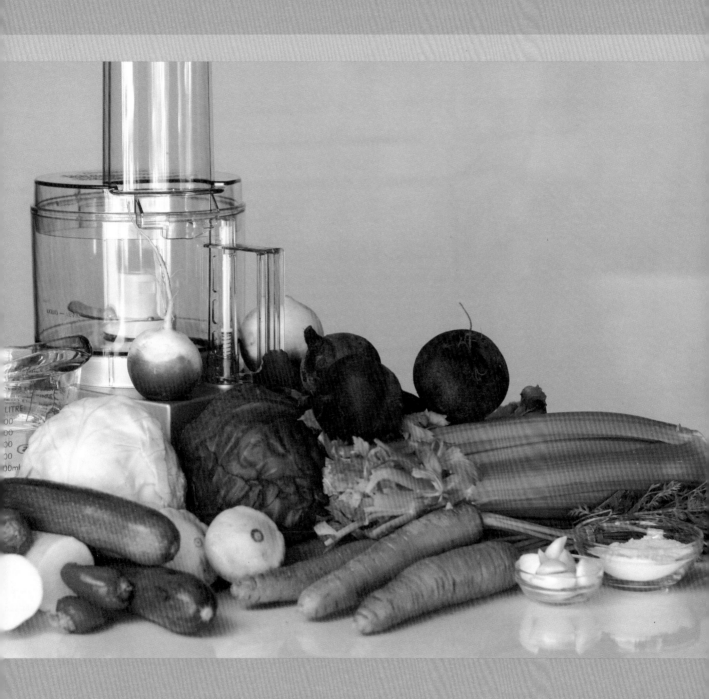

Cultured Vegetables

Cultured Vegetables

One wonderful benefit of this recipe is that it can be made out of almost any vegetables. All the different colors and textures in this marinated dish play a part in making it delectably gourmet.

Equipment

Food processor
Blender
Large bowl
1-gallon glass jar
Small glass jar
Cutting board
Knife
Potato masher

Ingredients

To make 1 gallon of cultured veggies you will need approximately 5 pounds of the following vegetables in any combination:

Red cabbage, green cabbage, rutabagas, carrots, celery stalks, celeriac (celery root), parsnips, turnips, beets, zucchini, radishes, and cauliflower.

You will also need to add the following:

3 cups water
6 large cloves garlic
3 hot peppers (jalapeño or other)
3 tbsp. salt (optional)
1 pkg. kefir or yoghurt culture (These are more commonly found in health-food stores. You can make the recipe without a culture; it will just take about 20 hours longer.)

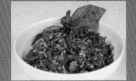

Most recipes for cultured veggies ask for large quantities of salt, because salt makes cabbage yield juice. Juice is necessary to submerge the fermenting vegetables so they are not exposed to the air and harmful microbes. Instead of using a lot of salt, we prepare a marinade by blending vegetables with water. You may also add herbs or spices to this liquid if you wish.

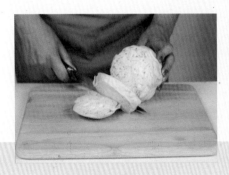 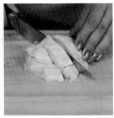 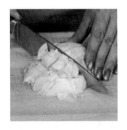 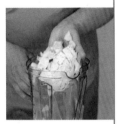

Rough-chop a quarter head of cabbage and add the cabbage pieces to the blender.

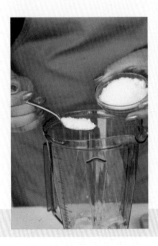 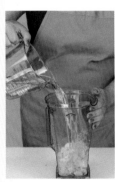 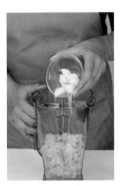

Add the salt, water, garlic, and kefir culture.

47

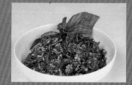
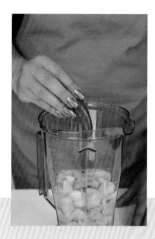

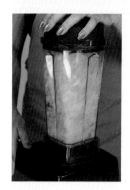

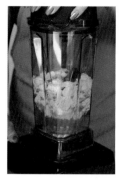

Add hot peppers and blend the mixture until it is smooth and has a pale green color. Set aside.

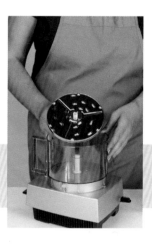

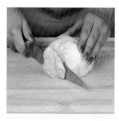

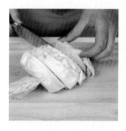

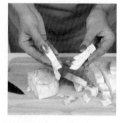

Position a grating blade in your food processor. Cut half a cabbage into pieces that will fit through the opening in the lid, about 1 inch wide.

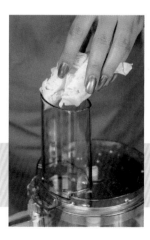

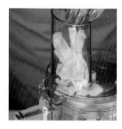

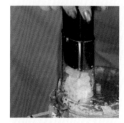

Begin shredding the cabbage by pushing it through the grater blade. You can grate the entire cabbage, leaves and stem.

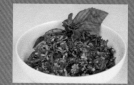

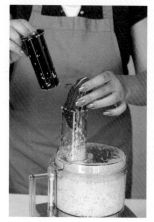
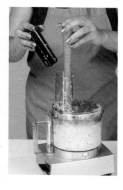
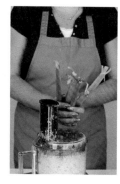
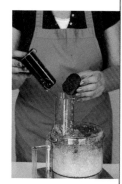

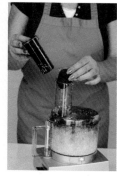
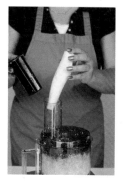
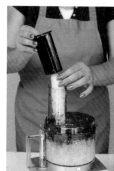

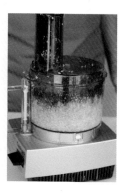

Celeriac (celery root) is an exceptionally tasty and nutritiously valuable vegetable. It has a soft, delicate texture and is even more nutritious than celery. It is rich in potassium, sodium, and vitamin C. Once you discover this delicious root, you will want to eat it regularly. We love to add grated celeriac to our salads. Celeriac is an excellent addition to any cultured food. It enhances the taste of your marinated veggies and increases their nutritional value.

Grate the other vegetables of your choice. Our favorite veggies are carrots, celery, parsnips, turnips, rutabagas, beets, zucchini, radishes, celery root, and cauliflower.

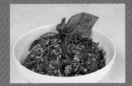

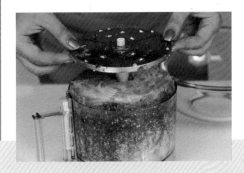 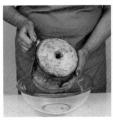 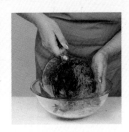 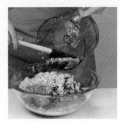

As you finish blending each batch, place the grated vegetables in a large bowl. You will fill your food processor's container several times over.

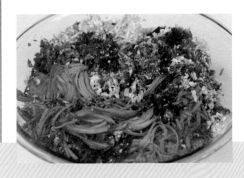 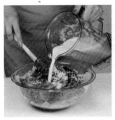 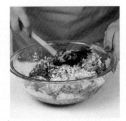 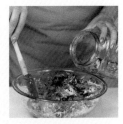

Begin to mix the beautiful colored vegetables together. Pour the cabbage marinade you made earlier into the mixed veggies and continue to stir.

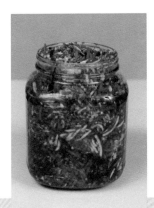 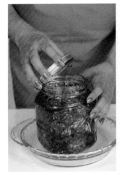

Transfer the mixed veggies into a glass gallon jar. Use a potato masher to compress the vegetables and cover them in their juice. Make sure there are no air pockets in order to prevent harmful microbes from growing. Press down hard on the shredded vegetables so all the air bubbles escape.

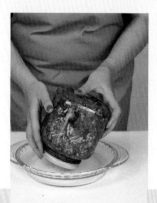

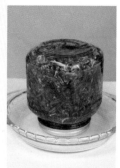

Put the lid on tightly and let the jar sit upside down for 2 to 3 hours so the juice has a chance to thoroughly penetrate the veggies in the jar.

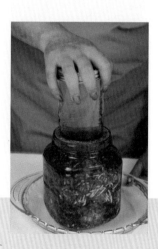

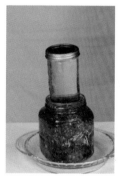

Find a small glass jar that will fit loosely into the mouth of the large jar to weigh down the vegetables. Fill it with water, put a lid on it, and place it in the large jar over the grated vegetables. Make sure there is a little space between the jars so that the air bubbles that rise from the mixture have room to escape.

Leave the jar out on your counter for 1 to 3 days. The longer you let the mixture sit, the more it will ferment.

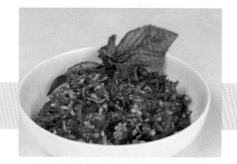

Serve cultured veggies sprinkled with oil and decorated with fresh herbs.

I remember how I couldn't convince my husband to help me make live garden burgers. Igor was afraid to spoil the ingredients. He reasoned, "It was easy with real meat; you just cut a piece and fried it with oil. But now I am supposed to create 'meat' from carrots, and without a cow?" He saw me preparing live garden burgers dozens of times, but he was certain that it was too complicated for him. One day, we had an emergency situation when too many people showed up for a catered raw food dinner. I was busy preparing soup. Somebody had to prepare garden burgers, and Igor didn't have a choice. So he did it! Even before I finished making soup, he was done. Since that day I have never made another live garden burger myself because Igor took over this task. Now in my family we call this dish "Igorburger."

Igor began to enjoy preparing raw food more and more. He created many of his own recipes. His Russian-style crackers are popular all over the world. In Iceland, Igor demonstrated how to prepare a raw sandwich. He put live garden burgers on crackers and decorated them with green leaves and tomatoes. When people tried his raw sandwiches they were amazed at how delicious they were. One woman exclaimed: "This sandwich is worth living for!"

We have perfected the live garden burger recipe throughout the years and are delighted to present it to you here in detail.

(Excerpt from the book *12 Steps to Raw Foods* by Victoria Boutenko. Please note: the recipe for the cracker mentioned above is also listed in this book on page 17.)

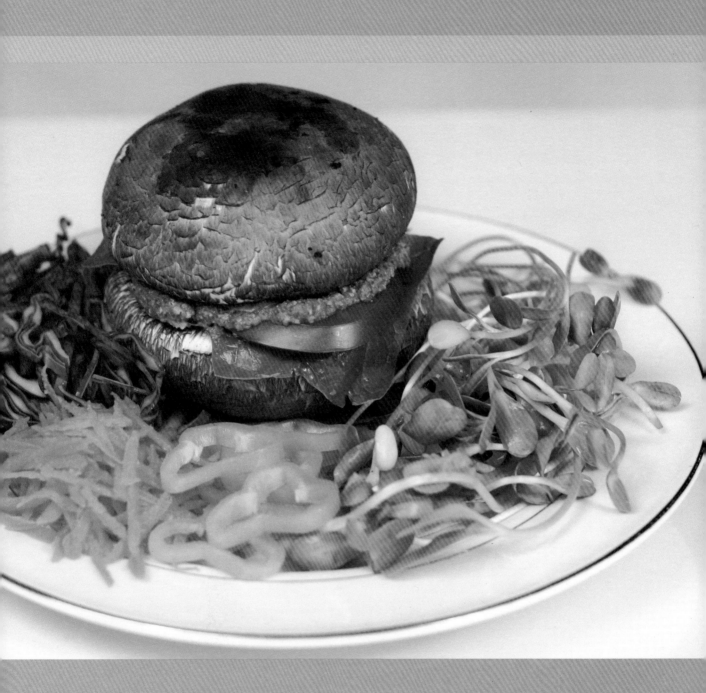

Live Garden Burger

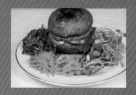

Live Garden Burger

You will find this delicious garden burger pâté is extremely versatile. Once you have the basic mixture together, you can build a traditional-style burger with mushroom patties (Portabella Burgers, pg. 59), try a cracker-based creation (Mini Pizzas, pg. 62), or get a little more fanciful (Bell Pepper Sailboat and Mushroom Fleet, pg. 63).

Equipment

Blender
Food processor
Citrus juicer
Bowl
Wooden spoon
Spatula
Cutting board
Knife
Ice-cream scoop

Ingredients

2 cups sunflower seeds
3 carrots
1 medium onion
¼ cup raisins
2 tbsp. raw agave nectar
¼ cup olive oil
1 lemon
¼ bunch fresh herbs (such as basil, thyme, dill, or rosemary)
1 tsp. sea salt
1 hot pepper (jalapeño or other)

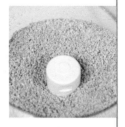

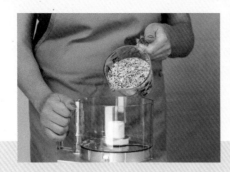
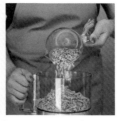
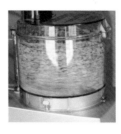

Put the S-blade in the food processor. Pour the sunflower seeds in the processor, secure the lid, and grind them to a powder.

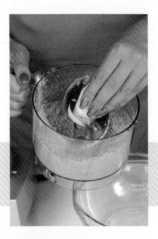
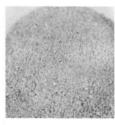
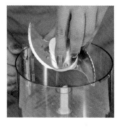

Remove the blade. Using the spatula, pour the powdered sunflower seeds into the bowl. Put the S-blade back into the processor.

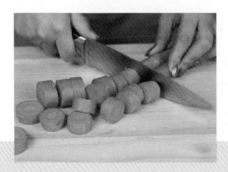
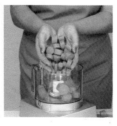
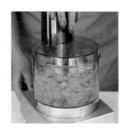
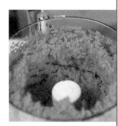

Cut the carrots into small chunks, approximately 1 inch thick, and add them to the food processor. Grind until they are pureed.

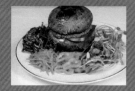
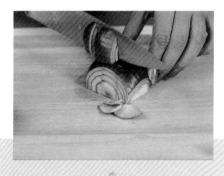
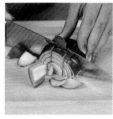
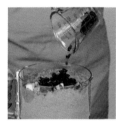

Slice the onion into small square pieces and add to the food processor.

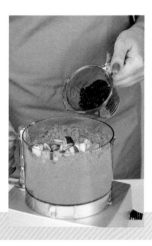
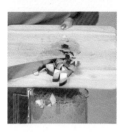
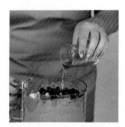

Add the raisins, raw agave nectar, and olive oil.

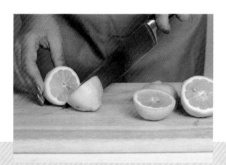
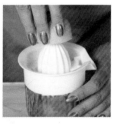
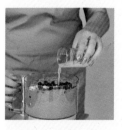

Slice the lemons in half, juice them, and pour the juice into the food processor.

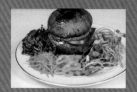

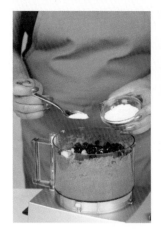

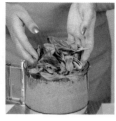

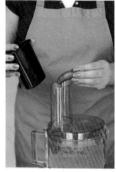

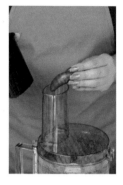

Add the sea salt, fresh herbs, and hot pepper. Blend the ingredients for approximately 1 minute.

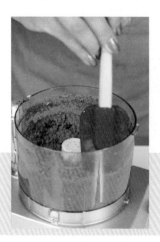

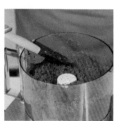

Stop blending, open the lid, and use a spatula to scrape down the contents from the walls of the container to ensure that the pâté is evenly blended throughout. Secure the lid and blend for another 30 seconds.

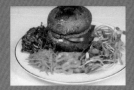
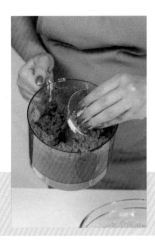

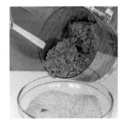

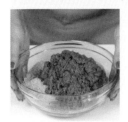

Take off the lid and remove the blade. Using the spatula, add the garden burger pâté to the bowl with the ground sunflower seeds.

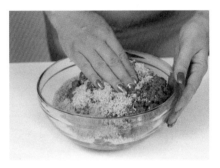

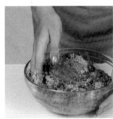

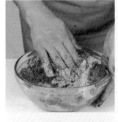

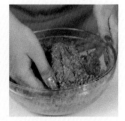

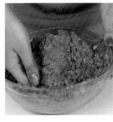

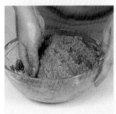

Knead the garden burger pâté with both hands until it is thoroughly mixed.

Now you have a bowl of delicious and nutritious garden burger pâté! We invite you to serve it as you would any burger or pâté. You can form it into balls, cutlets, or fillets and sprinkle with a little paprika. We offer several ideas below; you may come up with unlimited variations of your own.

This recipe makes roughly 4 cups of pâté, enough for about 4 portabella burgers, 10 pizzas, or 6 bell pepper sailboats. It will keep in the refrigerator for several days so you can use it for a variety of dishes during the week.

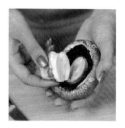

Portabella Burgers

For this recipe, pick out firm, evenly shaped portabella mushrooms—two for each burger.

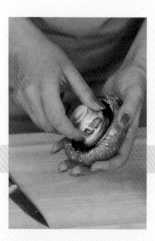
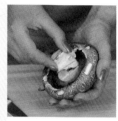
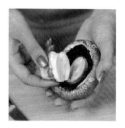

Carefully cut out the mushroom stalks.

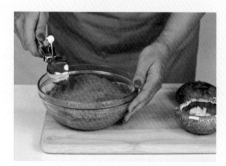
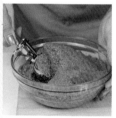
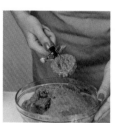
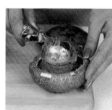
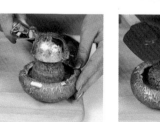
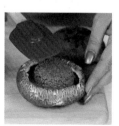
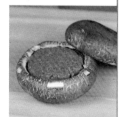

With the ice-cream scoop, portion out a burger from the pâté and place it on the flat side of the mushroom. Flatten the burger with the spatula.

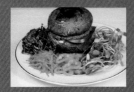
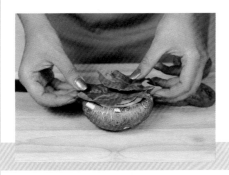

Cut a thin slice of onion and add it on top of the burger.

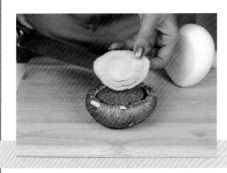

Layer a couple of bright green leaves of lettuce or spinach.

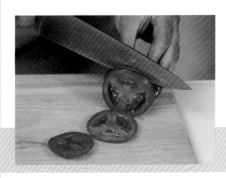

Cut a couple of thin slices of tomato and place them on the green leaves.

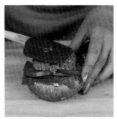

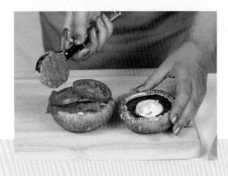

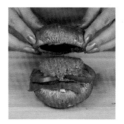

Scoop out another burger and add it on top of the tomatoes. Flatten the burger with the spatula.

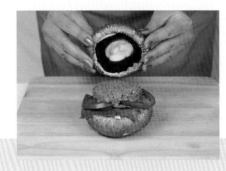

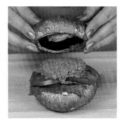

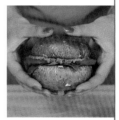

Add more green leaves to the burger and top off your sandwich with another mushroom "bun."

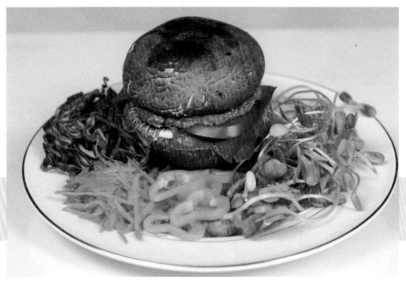

Serve your mushroom burger with a variety of veggies and sprouts.

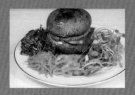

Mini Pizzas

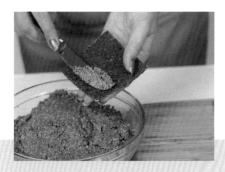 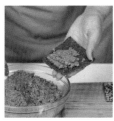 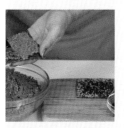

Using a butter knife, spread a layer of garden burger pâté on a few crackers (see our recipe on page 17.)

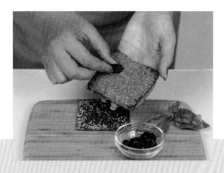 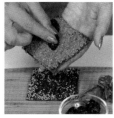 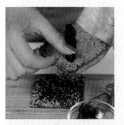

Decorate as you wish, with sun-dried olives, sliced mushrooms, halved cherry tomatoes, herbs, and other vegetables.

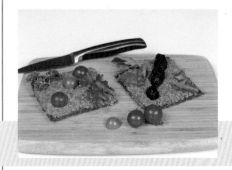

These charming personal-size pizzas are very satisfying as a main course, or can make perfect appetizers for guests.

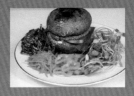

Bell Pepper Sailboat and Mushroom Fleet

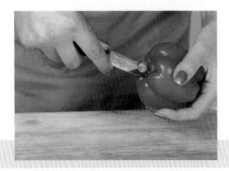

Remove the stem, seeds, and core from a bell pepper.

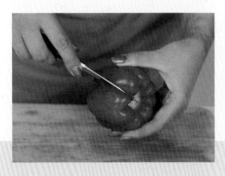 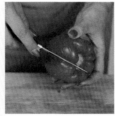

Cut the pepper in half, sideways along the grooves. This way you will have two parts, each resembling the hull of a boat. Remove any extra seeds.

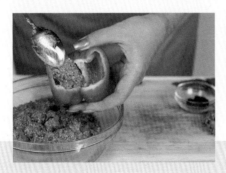 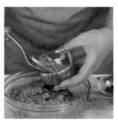

Using a spoon, fill each half with garden burger pâté. Smooth down the filling to look like a deck.

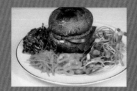
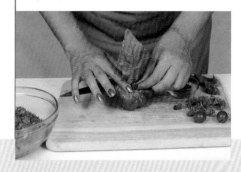

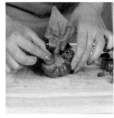

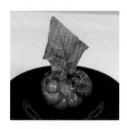

Stick a big spinach or basil leaf up in the middle to look like a sail. Decorate with your favorite veggies and herbs. You may serve your sailboats alone, or you can add a mushroom fleet!

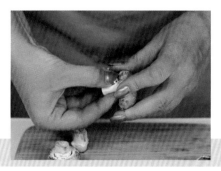

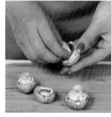

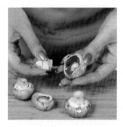

Carefully twist off the stalks from the button mushrooms.

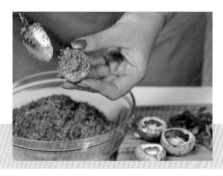

Using a spoon or small ice-cream scoop, fill the mushrooms with pâté.

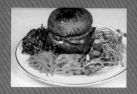

Decorate with whole cherry tomatoes and herbs.

Our family has served this fun and pretty dish at children's parties, weddings, birthdays, and many other festive gatherings.

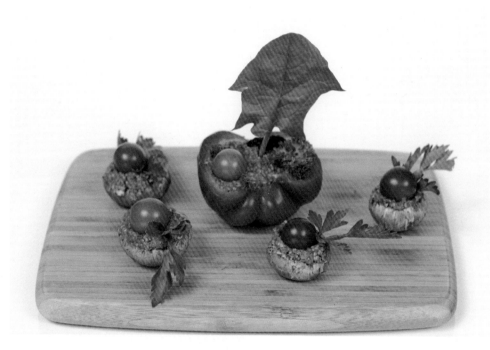

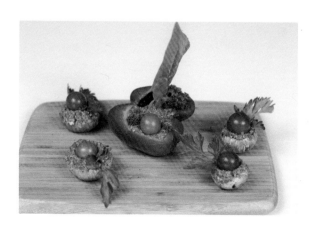

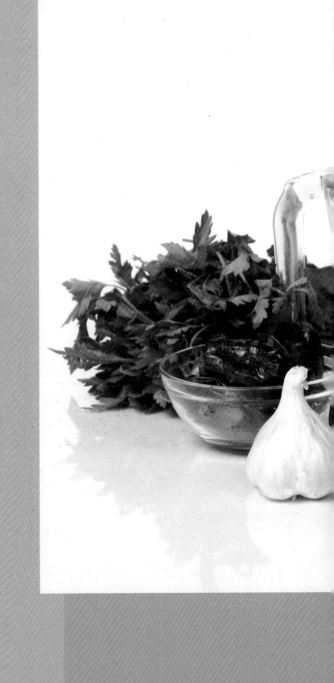

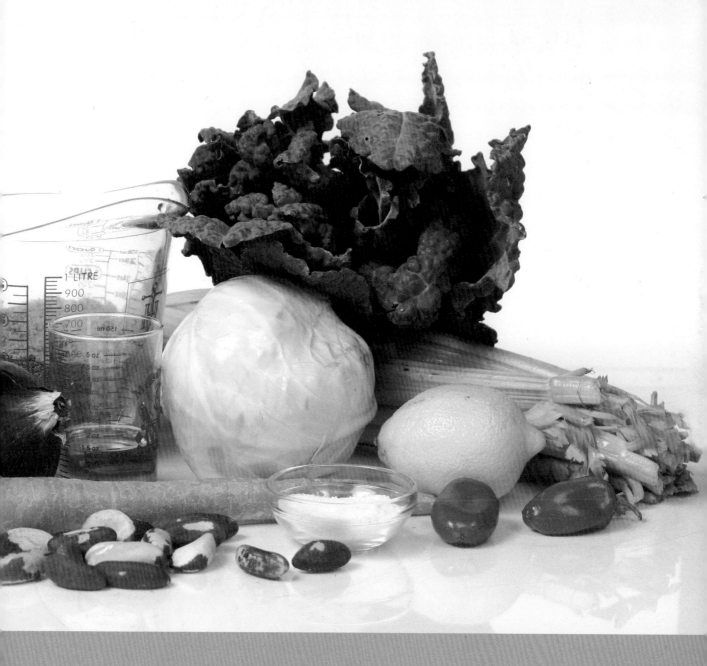

Peroshkis

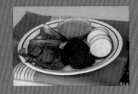

Peroshkis

Peroshkis, or pierogies, are to Russians what pizza is to Italians. We missed peroshkis when we came from Russia. We missed peroshkis even more hopelessly when we went on the raw food diet. In an effort to convince our Russian friends of the benefits of eating raw, we experimented until we were able to re-create this famous Russian dish. Everybody who tries them enjoys them, no matter what their diet. Now that we are in love with greens, we offer you a recipe of peroshkis with kale. (Green eggs and ham will be in the next book!)

Equipment

Dehydrator
Vita-Mix blender or
    coffee grinder
Food processor
Large bowl
Ice-cream scoop
Cutting board
Knife
Spatula
Citrus juicer

Ingredients

2 pounds celery (about 1 large bunch)
2 pounds cabbage (1 medium-sized cabbage)
2 large carrots
2 tbsp. extra-virgin olive oil (optional)
6–9 dates, pits removed
3 tbsp. sea salt (optional)
2 jalapeños, or other hot peppers
5 cloves garlic
1 medium onion
6 medium lemons
2 bunches kale
1 pound Brazil nuts (or sunflower seeds)
2 bunches parsley or cilantro
1 lb. flaxseed, ground in a coffee grinder or a Vita-Mix
3 tbsp. paprika powder

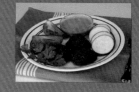

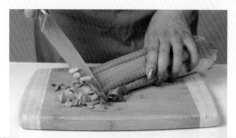
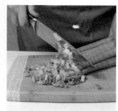

Slice celery into 1-inch chunks.

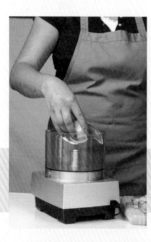
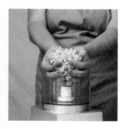
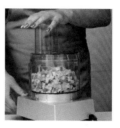

Position the S-blade in the food processor. Fill the container approximately halfway full with chopped celery. Grind well.

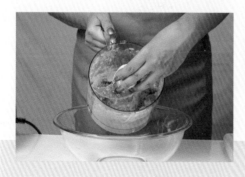
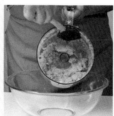

Remove the blade and use a spatula to scoop the ground celery into a large bowl. Repeat as necessary until all celery is ground.

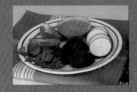
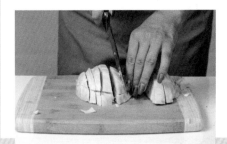 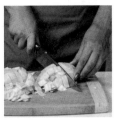

Cut a head of cabbage in half. Chop up both halves into approximately 1-inch squares.

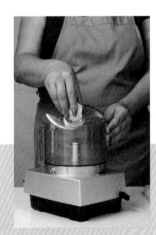 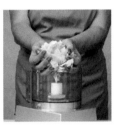

Position the S-blade in the food processor, fill the container approximately halfway full with chopped cabbage, and blend. Remove the blade and use a spatula to scoop the ground cabbage into the bowl with celery. Repeat until most of the cabbage is ground, saving some to grind with the carrots so your processor is full enough to work efficiently.

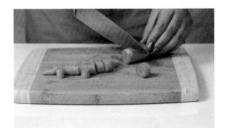 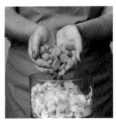

Place the last remaining batch of cabbage in the food processor. Chop the carrots into approximately 1-inch rounds and add them to the food processor on top of the cabbage.

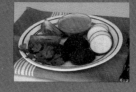

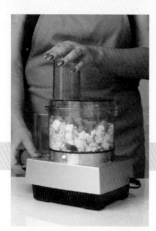

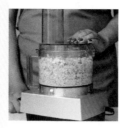

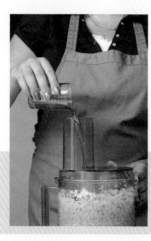

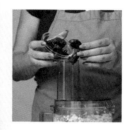

Grind thoroughly.

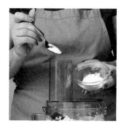

Add the extra virgin olive oil, dates (make sure all pits are removed), and salt. (The oil helps with consistency, but is not absolutely necessary, and you may omit the salt as well if you prefer.)

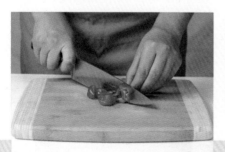

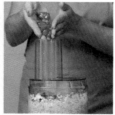

Add jalapeños. You may add more than two peppers if you like spicy food.

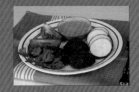
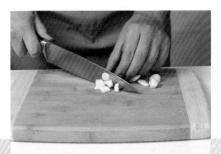

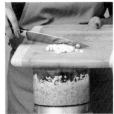

Peel and chop the garlic cloves and add them to the processor.

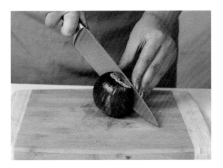

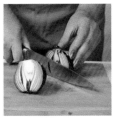

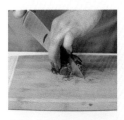

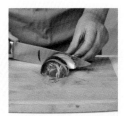

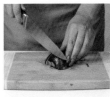

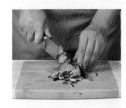

Peel and chop the onion.

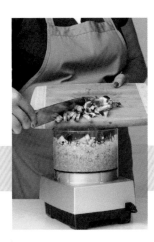

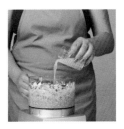

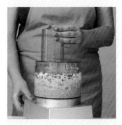

Add onion and lemon juice to the processor and grind thoroughly.

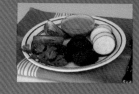

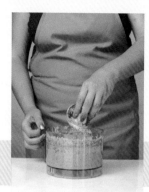
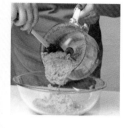
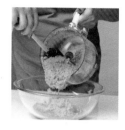

Remove the blade and use a spatula to scoop the mixture into the bowl with the other ground veggies.

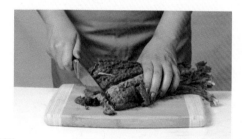
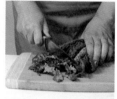
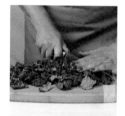

Rough-chop two bunches of kale.

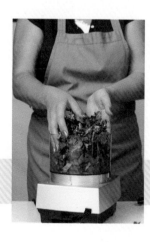
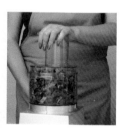

Fill the whole processor container with chopped kale. Grind well and repeat until all kale is pureed.

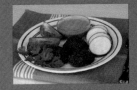
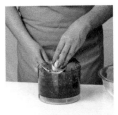
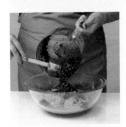

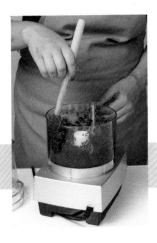

Remove the blade and use a spatula to scoop out the kale and add it to the bowl with the other ground vegetables.

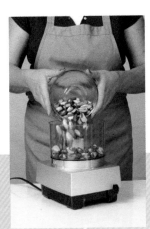
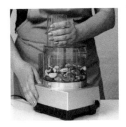

Fill the food processor halfway with Brazil nuts. Grind them thoroughly until they turn into a flour. (Please note: if you grind them too long, they might turn into a nut butter.)

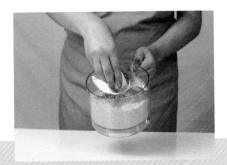
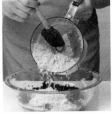

Remove the blade and use a spatula to scoop the ground nuts into the bowl of vegetables. Repeat until most of the Brazil nuts are ground.

Place the remaining nuts in the food processor. Grind well, and leave them in the container while you prep the kale.

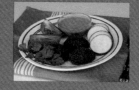

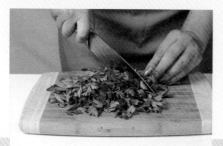
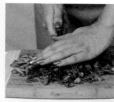
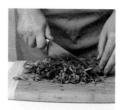

Rough-chop two bunches of parsley.

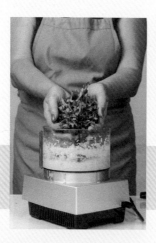
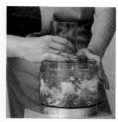
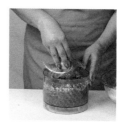
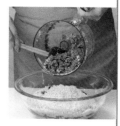

Add them to the processor with the nuts and grind. Remove the blade and use a spatula to scoop the ground nuts and parsley into the bowl of ground vegetables.

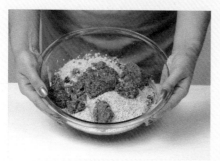
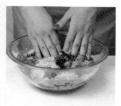
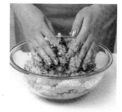
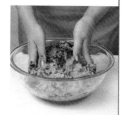

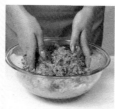

Knead the dough thoroughly with your hands.

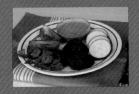
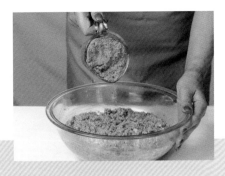
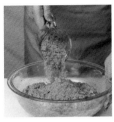
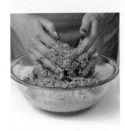

Add the ground flaxseed to the dough, and mix it in well with your hands.

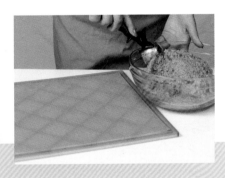
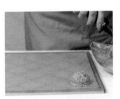

Prepare dehydrator trays by placing a sheet of mesh plastic on each of them, and add a Teflex or other nonstick sheet over the mesh.

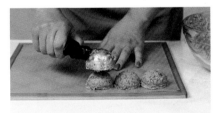
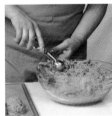
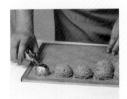
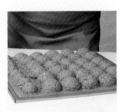

Using an ice-cream scoop, scoop mounds of dough onto the tray. (Any spoon will do, but the scoop helps give the peroshkis a more uniform shape.)

You can place the peroshkis very close together as they will shrink while drying. Make even rows so they dry evenly.

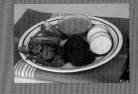

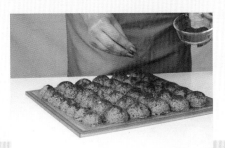

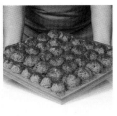

Once the tray is filled, sprinkle paprika on the peroshkis for a more attractive appearance.

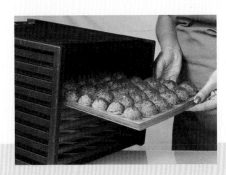

Dehydrate at 105 to 115 degrees F for approximately 15 to 20 hours, depending on the temperature and humidity of your kitchen. You may want to remove the Teflex sheets after about 12 hours and leave your peroshkis on mesh sheets for more thorough drying.

Peroshkis taste best when fresh, but you can store them in the refrigerator for several weeks.

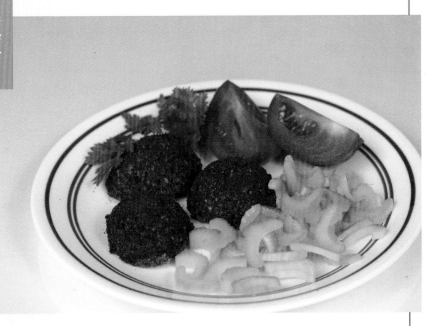

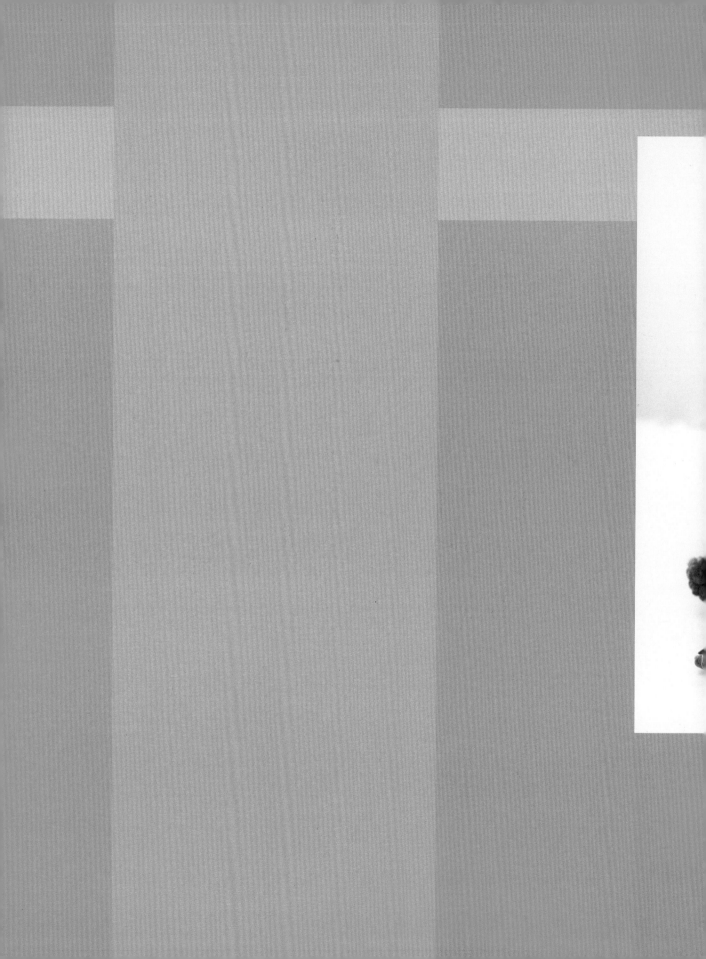

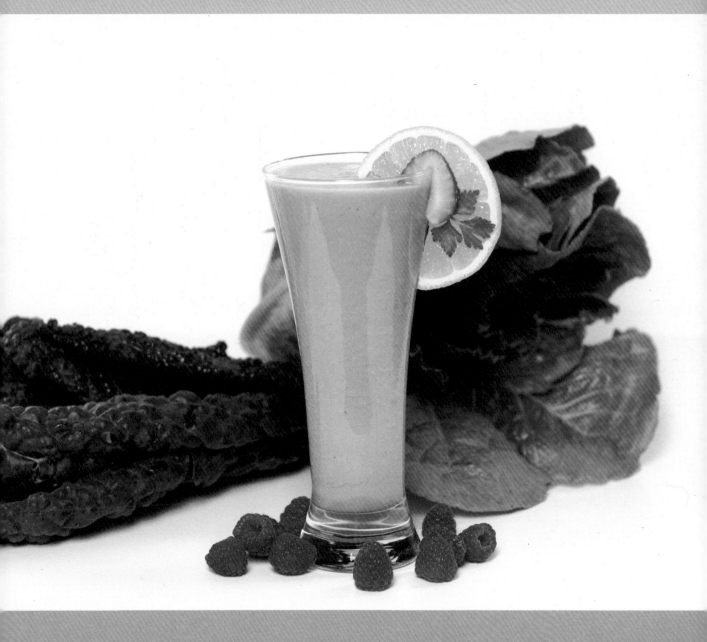

Green Smoothie

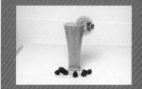

Green Smoothie

We drink green smoothies every day because we consider them to be the most nutritious food in the world. Through many years of research, we have learned that greens are a prime source of nutrition. They are rich in essential vitamins, minerals, amino acids, and antioxidants. Adding ripe fruit to green smoothies makes even the most bitter greens palatable. We enjoy green smoothies so much that we bought an extra blender and placed it in the Raw Family office so we can make green smoothies any time. We share them with everyone who comes in. Even our FedEx driver loves green smoothies!

Equipment

Blender
Cutting board
Knife

Ingredients

1 pineapple
2 mangoes
1 bunch chard
2 cups water

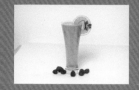

Green smoothies have numerous benefits for human health.

1. Green smoothies are very nutritious. The ratio of about 60 percent ripe, organic fruit mixed with about 40 percent organic green leaves is optimal for human consumption.

2. Green smoothies are easy to digest. When blended well, most of the cells in the greens and fruits are ruptured, making the valuable nutrients easy for the body to assimilate. Green smoothies literally start to get absorbed in your mouth.

3. Green smoothies, as opposed to juices, are a complete food because they still have fiber. Consuming fiber is important for our elimination system.

4. Those who eat a standard American diet enjoy the taste of green smoothies because the fruit taste dominates the flavor, yet at the same time the greens balance out the sweetness of the fruit, adding a nice zest to it. People trying green smoothies for the first time are usually quite surprised that something so green could taste so nice.

5. A molecule of chlorophyll closely resembles a molecule of human blood. According to the teachings of Dr. Ann Wigmore, consuming chlorophyll is like receiving a healthy blood transfusion. Many people do not consume enough greens—even those on a raw food diet. By drinking two or three cups of green smoothie a day you will consume enough greens to nourish your body, and all of the beneficial nutrients will be well assimilated.

6. Green smoothies are easy to make, and quick to clean up after. In contrast, juicing greens is time consuming, messy, and expensive. Many people abandon drinking green juices on a regular basis for those reasons. Preparing a pitcher of green smoothie takes less than 5 minutes, including cleaning.

7. Green smoothies are loved by children of all ages, including babies of 6 or more months old. Of course you have to be careful and slowly increase the amount of smoothie to avoid food allergies.

8. When consuming your greens in the form of green smoothies, you are greatly reducing the consumption of oils and salt in your diet.

9. Regular consumption of green smoothies forms a good habit of eating greens. After a few weeks of drinking green smoothies, most people start to enjoy and crave eating more greens. Eating enough greens is often a problem with many people, especially children.

10. While fresh is always best, green smoothies will keep in cool temperatures for up to 3 days, which can be handy at work and while traveling.

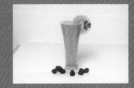
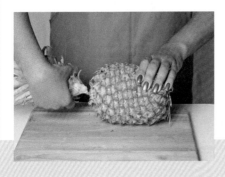
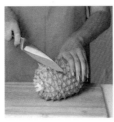
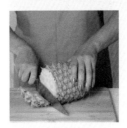

Remove the stem of the pineapple by gripping the fruit firmly and twisting the top off. Cut approximately one inch off the bottom and the top.

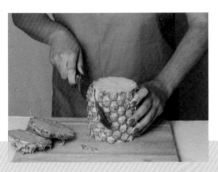
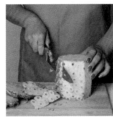
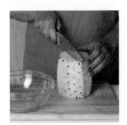

Slice off the prickly skin of the pineapple and cut the fruit in slices approximately ½ inch thick. Make sure all the coarse pieces of skin are removed. There may still be some dark dots but they can be blended into the smoothie.

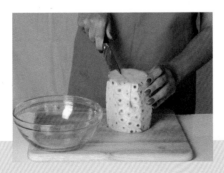
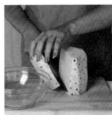
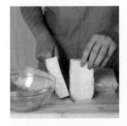
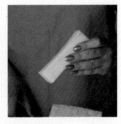

If you have a high-speed blender such as Vita-Mix or Blendtec, you do not have to remove the core of the pineapple. If you have a regular blender, you will need to remove the core. To remove the core, cut the flesh off the pineapple, working the knife closely around the core.

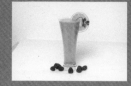

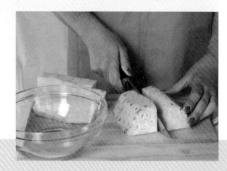 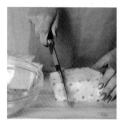 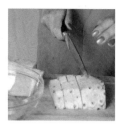 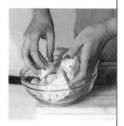

Cut the rest of the pineapple into chunks, place them in a bowl, and set aside.

You may place the pineapple core in the refrigerator and use it later. You can chop it into cubes and enjoy it as a snack, or (if you have a high-speed blender) juice it with other ingredients, which will add a nice tropical flavor to your fruit or vegetable juice.

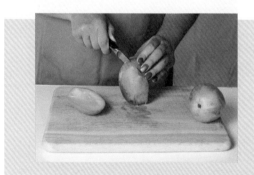

There are many different ways to cut mangoes. We will teach you our family favorite.

Keep in mind that inside the mango is a thin, flat pit. Starting at the top, make a lengthwise cut as close to the pit as possible. Make a similar cut on the other side.

Now you have two halves of mango, which contain most of the flesh. Set aside the middle section containing the pit. You can eat around what's left on the seed or compost it.

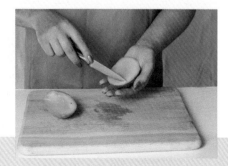 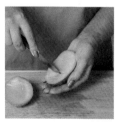 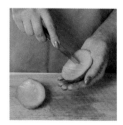 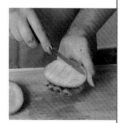

Holding one half of the mango in your palm, gently make a grid of cuts with a small paring knife by first cutting one direction, then across, close to the bottom skin without puncturing it. Be very careful not to cut your hand.

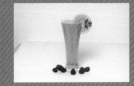
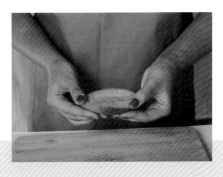 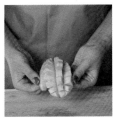

Holding the mango with both hands, turn the mango inside out to fan out the chunks.

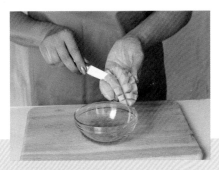 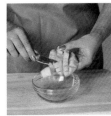 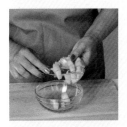 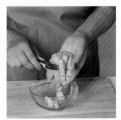

It is now easy to cut the chunks off into a bowl. Prepare the three other mango halves in the same way.

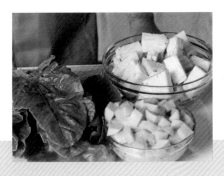 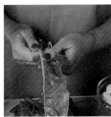

Next, prepare the chard. The entire chard plant is edible, but we like to remove the stems because they add a salty or peppery taste to the smoothie, and they don't blend well in a regular blender.

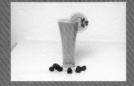

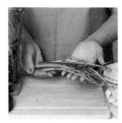

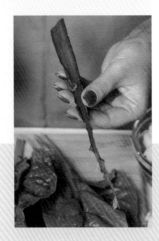

To remove stems, hold the stem in one hand and strip off the leaves with the other. Don't bother removing the smaller parts of the stem that don't naturally separate from the leaves; just the main stalk. You may chop up the stem later and add it to a salad.

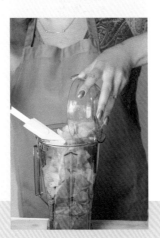

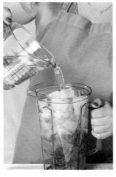

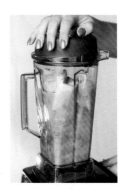

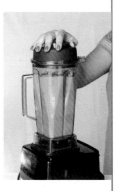

Place all the fruit and greens into the blender, add water, and secure the lid. Blend well to a creamy consistency.

This recipe makes a full blender's worth, approximately half a gallon of delicious green smoothie. Of course, drinking a smoothie fresh is optimal, but we often don't have time to make one right before we want to drink it. One of the benefits of green smoothies is that you can keep them in the refrigerator up to three days.

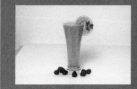
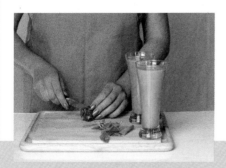

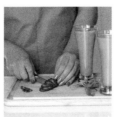

We invite you to serve the smoothie in pretty glasses and decorate it with fresh, brightly colored fruit.

There are unlimited varieties of green smoothies you could make. Every time you change the greens or add different fruit, you are creating an original recipe with a whole new flavor! (All greens contain a minute amount of alkaloids. If you consume the same greens for many weeks, you can accumulate the alkaloid, so rotate them daily, for example kale on Monday, spinach on Tuesday, and so on.)

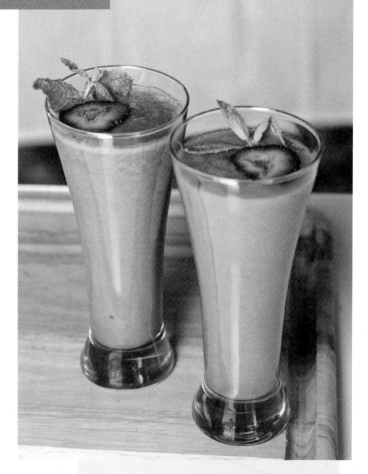

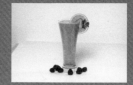

Here are a few more of our family's favorite smoothie recipes:

Minty Sweet Spinach

1 bunch spinach
1 sprig of mint
1 pint strawberries
3 ripe bananas
2 cups water

Blend all ingredients until smooth. Yields 2 quarts of smoothie.

Tooth of the Lion Smoothie

The word "dandelion" comes from the old French, dent de lion, "tooth of (a) lion." Centuries ago people noticed that those who consumed dandelion leaves had teeth as strong as lions. (Source: http://dictionary.reference.com/browse/dandelion)

1 bunch dandelion leaves
2 mangoes
2 pears
2 cups water

Blend all ingredients until smooth. Yields 2 quarts of smoothie.

Peachy Green

1 bunch kale, destemmed
4 ripe peaches
2 cups water

Blend all ingredients until smooth. Yields 2 quarts of smoothie.

These recipes are merely basic ideas for your green creations. Feel free to substitute the ingredients with your own choice of greens and fruits. Enjoy!

Start playing with green smoothies, and discover the many joys and benefits of this wonderful delicious and nutritious addition to your menu. You may find many more amazing facts about green smoothies in my books *Green for Life* and *Green Smoothie Revolution*.

Nuts and seeds are nutritionally dense foods, as well as delicious in nut milks. Our all-time favorite nut milks are almond and sesame seed. Here is some impressive information about these two seeds.

Almonds

Almonds are extremely rich in vitamin E and B as well as riboflavin, niacin, thiamin, and folate. Almonds are high in Omega-6.

One cup of almonds contains 40 percent of the U.S. RDA of protein, while a cup of low-fat cow's milk contains just 16 percent.

Almonds are high in the following minerals: manganese, magnesium, calcium, iron, copper, zinc, potassium, and phosphorus.

Sesame Seeds

One cup of sesame seeds (unhulled) has 140 percent of the U.S. RDA of calcium and 116 percent of the U.S. RDA of iron, as well as 294 percent of the requirement for copper. It is also high in manganese, magnesium, and zinc. Sesame seeds are rich in B vitamins and Omega-6.

Source: www.nutritiondata.com. The information in this database comes from the USDA's National Nutrient Database for Standard Reference.

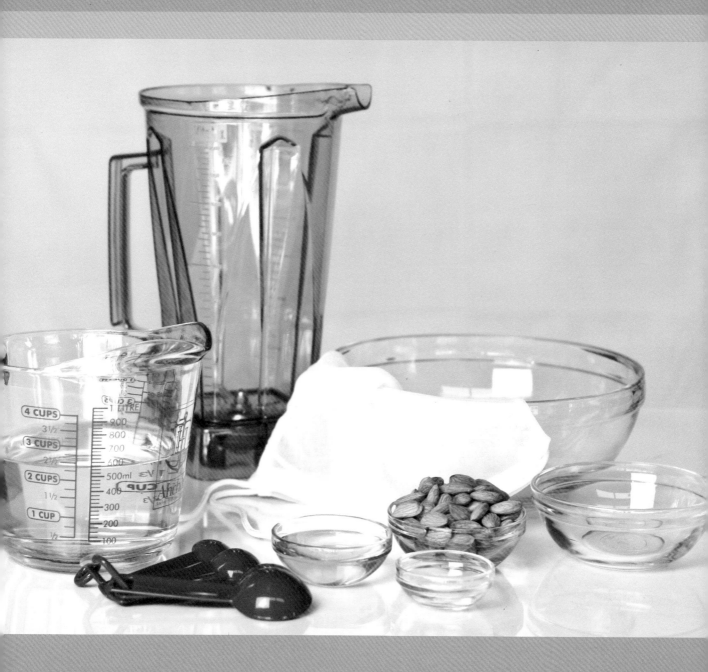

Nut Milk

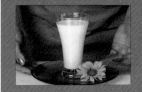

Nut Milk

Nut milks are a miraculously simple food to prepare, and will quickly become an everyday favorite. It is so comforting to cuddle up with a blanket, a good book, and a cup of nut milk after a long stressful day.

There are unlimited variations on this basic nut milk recipe. In our family, we've enjoyed nut milks hundreds of times, yet they always taste slightly different and continue to surprise us with their wonderful flavor.

To prepare a nut milk, you will need:

Equipment
Blender
Nut-milk bag
Large bowl
Small bowl for soaking
   nuts, and later for nut
    pulp
Pitcher

Ingredients
1 cup almonds
3 cups water
3 tbsp. raw agave nectar
⅛ tsp. sea salt (optional)

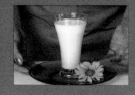

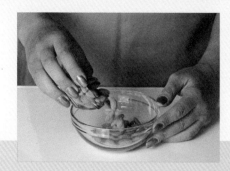

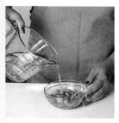

Pour the nuts into the small bowl and cover with water. Set the bowl aside for the night, or for about 6 hours.

We recommend that you always soak nuts or seeds overnight in water. Dry nuts and seeds contain enzyme inhibitors that are not good for the body. Soaking destroys the inhibitors and makes nuts more digestible.

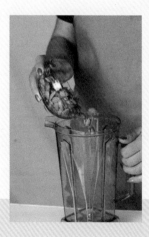

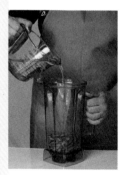

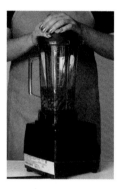

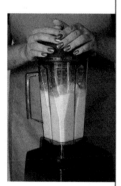

After the nuts have soaked, pour the leftover water out and place the nuts in the blender. Add three cups of fresh water, cover the blender securely, and blend well.

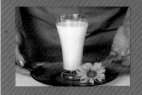
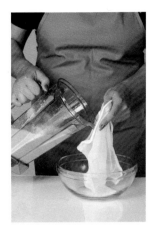
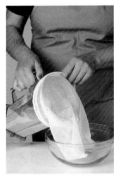
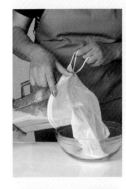
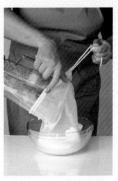
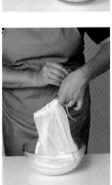
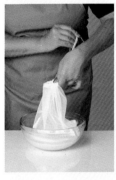
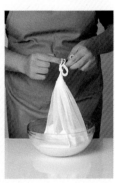
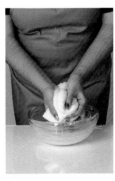
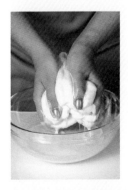

Over a large bowl, pour the mixture into the nut-milk bag and tie the bag tight.

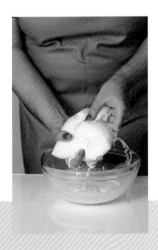

As you squeeze the milk through the bag, make sure to use both hands so that the pressure from your hands is spread evenly, which will prevent the bag from splitting at the seam.

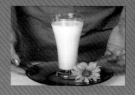

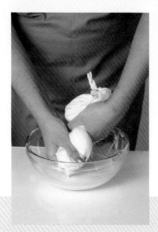
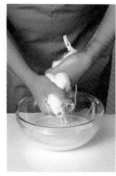

Gently squeeze the nut-milk bag, alternating pressure between your right and left hands. Keep squeezing until the bag is completely drained, and only the pulp is left inside.

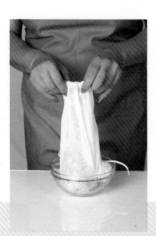
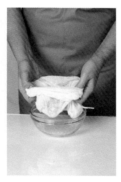
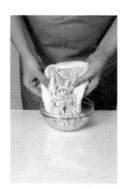
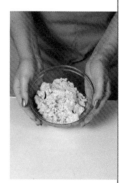

Carefully open the bag over the small bowl and pour out the pulp. (You may store the pulp in the freezer for an indefinite amount of time and use it later for other recipes.)

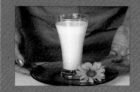

You can come up with an unlimited variety of flavors in your nut milks by changing the ingredients. Try experimenting with the following nuts and seeds: almonds, hazelnuts, Brazil nuts, pecans, macadamia nuts, walnuts, pine nuts, pistachios, pumpkin seeds, hemp seeds, sunflower seeds, or sesame seeds.

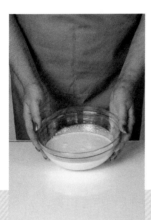
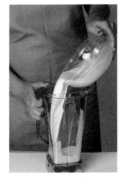
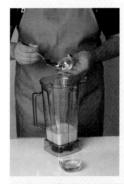
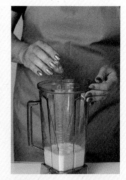

If you like, you can drink the nut milk as it is. Some people prefer its very mild flavor. To add a more distinctive flavor, pour the milk back into the blender, add the agave nectar and salt, and blend the mixture for just 10 or 15 seconds.

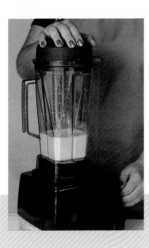
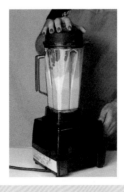
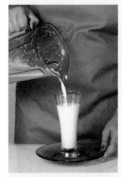

The nut milk may become slightly warm from blending, which is comforting on a cold, rainy day. In the summer you may enjoy your nut milk chilled.

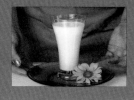

You may add a pinch of one of the following spices to your nut milk: nutmeg, vanilla, cinnamon, allspice, mint, or cloves.

And try the following sweeteners: agave nectar, dates, honey, stevia, raisins, bananas, or apple juice.

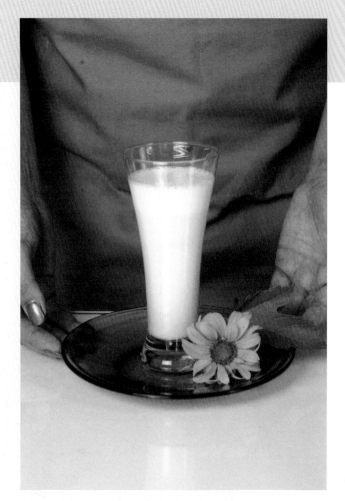

For special occasions, serve your guests nut milk with a bright flower or sprinkle some nuts around the glass.

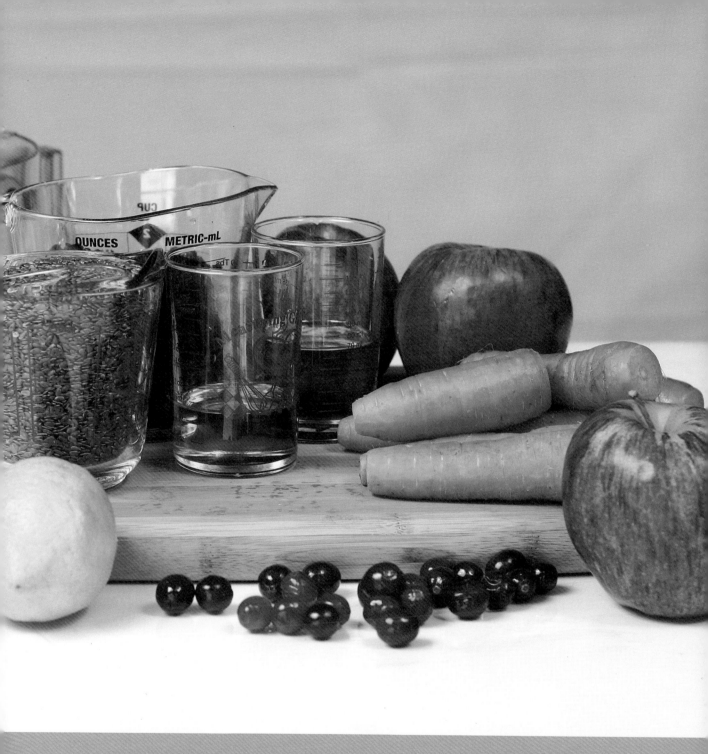

Cranberry Scones

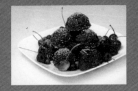
Cranberry Scones

Cranberry scones have a pleasant sweet-and-sour taste and a texture similar to bran muffins. Raw scones are not baked but dehydrated, and therefore keep all the nutrients intact. We like this recipe because it consists of more apples and carrots and fewer nuts. These scones make a hearty snack and are convenient for traveling.

Equipment

Food processor
Dehydrator
Citrus juicer
High-speed blender or
    coffee grinder
Cutting board
Knife
Large bowl
Ice-cream scoop
Spatula

Ingredients

2 cups grated carrots (about 2 carrots)
2 cups grated apples (about 2 apples)
2 cups walnuts
2 cups raisins
1 cup cranberries (fresh or frozen)
1 cup flaxseed
4 tbsp. raw agave nectar
¼ cup lemon juice
2 tbsp. olive oil
2 tbsp. sesame seeds, hulled or unhulled

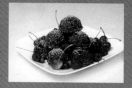

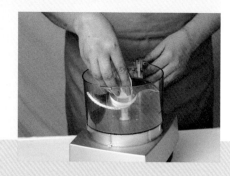 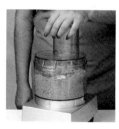

Put the S-blade into your processor. Slice carrots into approximately 1-inch chunks, put them into the processor, and grind them until they are a fine consistency.

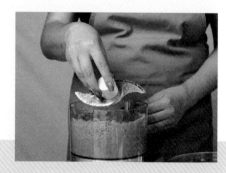 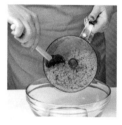

Remove the blade and using a spatula, pour the carrots into a large bowl.

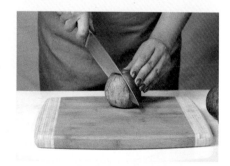 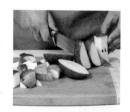 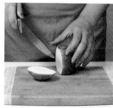 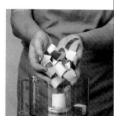

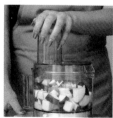 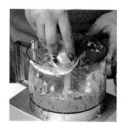

Put the S-blade back in the processor and repeat the same steps with the apples—slice into 1-inch chunks and grind them thoroughly. Take the blade out and pour the apples into the bowl with the carrots.

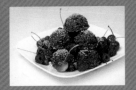
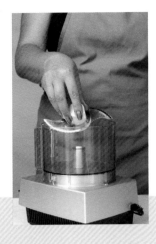

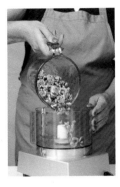

Before grinding the nuts, rinse and thoroughly dry your food processor with a towel or cloth so the nuts do not stick to the container.

Put the S-blade back in, add the walnuts to the processor, and grind well.

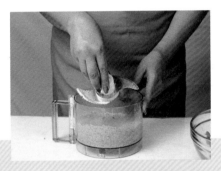

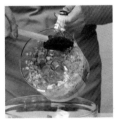

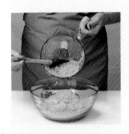

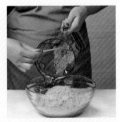

Take the blade out. Using a spatula, add the ground nuts to the mixing bowl.

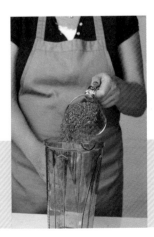

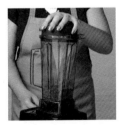

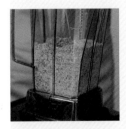

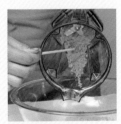

In a high-speed blender or coffee grinder, grind the flaxseed to a powder. Add the ground flaxseed to the mixing bowl. Use a spatula or chopstick to get all the ground flaxseed out of the container.

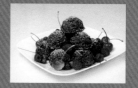

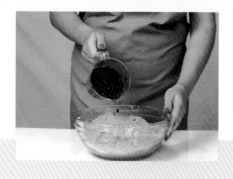
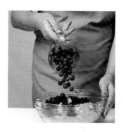
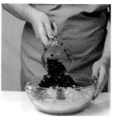
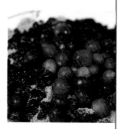

Add the raisins and cranberries to the mixture. Now you have a colorful mix that already begins to look yummy!

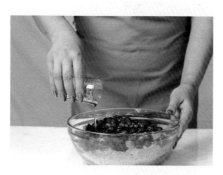
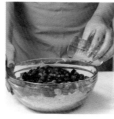
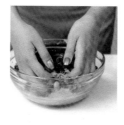
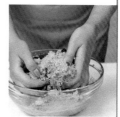
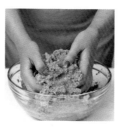
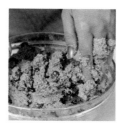
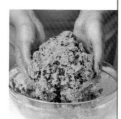

Pour the raw agave nectar, lemon juice, and olive oil into the bowl and start mixing the ingredients with both hands.
Keep mixing the dough until there are no chunks or dry pockets left.

We encourage you to think how happy your friends will be when you share the scones with them, or you may pray or meditate or sing. Japanese scientists have proven that the positive thinking of chefs enhances the nutritional value and taste of food.

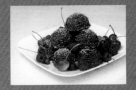
Place a Teflex or other nonstick sheet over the plastic mesh sheet on top of the dehydrator tray.

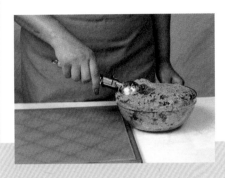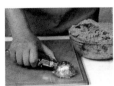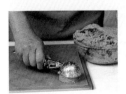

Using the ice-cream scoop, scoop mounds of dough onto the tray. (Any spoon will do, but the scoop helps make a more uniform shape for all the scones.)

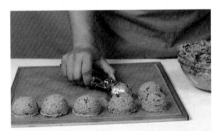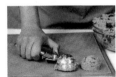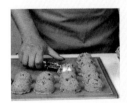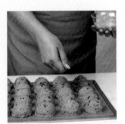

Position the scones close together as they will shrink while drying. Make uniform rows so that the scones dry evenly. Start with the far side first, or else rotate the tray.

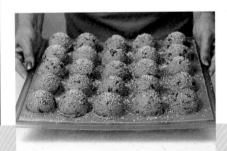

For an attractive finish, sprinkle sesame seeds on top of the scones.

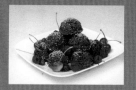

Dehydrate at 105 to 115 degrees F for approximately 15 to 20 hours, depending on the temperature and humidity in your kitchen, then flip the scones and dehydrate for another 3 hours on the opposite side.

The scones will keep in a glass or plastic container for up to 2 months in the refrigerator or for 2 weeks at room temperature.

Makes 25 scones.

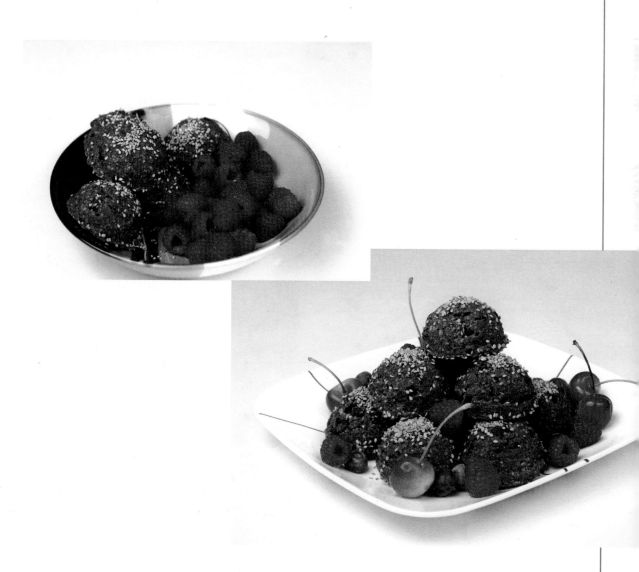

Raw jams closely resemble traditional jams in taste, flavor, and consistency, although raw jams are not cooked and therefore do not keep for long periods of time. Raw jams are much more nutritious than cooked jams and possess a number of other benefits that traditional jams do not.

Raw jams:

• have only half of the calories that regularly cooked jams do

• do not contain white sugar or any other sweetener

• are rich in natural vitamins, minerals, and antioxidants

• take just minutes to prepare and are one of the simplest recipes ever

• are a delicious treat for dessert lovers

• create a beautiful addition to a party table

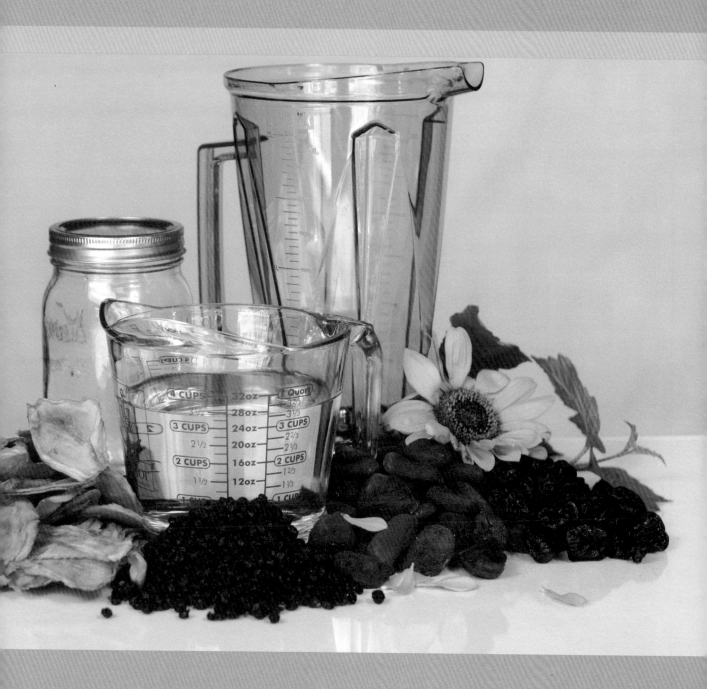

Raw Mango Jam

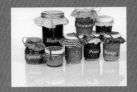

Raw Mango Jam

The following recipe may be used for making jam out of
any dried fruit. The quality of the dried fruit you use is
important. We like to use fruit that we have dried ourselves
during the harvest season, but we also buy quality dried
organic fruit from health-food stores. Be sure to avoid the
brands using sulfides.

Equipment

Blender
Small glass jar
Small bowl

Ingredients

2 cups dried mangoes
2 cups water

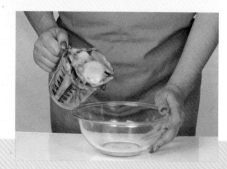 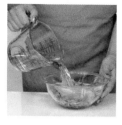 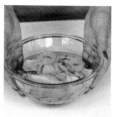

Soak dried mangoes in enough water to completely submerge them, about 2 cups. Leave them to soak for 15 to 20 minutes.

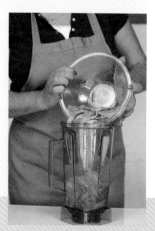 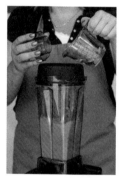 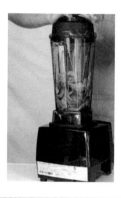 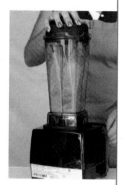

After 20 minutes, when the dried mangoes are slightly reconstituted, pour them and the soak water into a blender. Blend the mango pieces until smooth. The mango jam will become thicker as you blend it. If the jam becomes so thick that it stops circulating, add a small amount of water to the mixture.

Once the mango jam is blended, it should have a pleasant golden color and smell absolutely heavenly. Transfer the jam into a clean jar and store in the refrigerator.

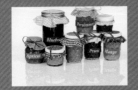

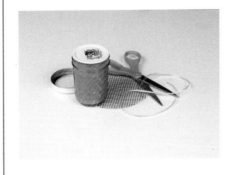 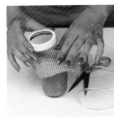 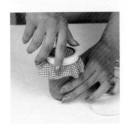 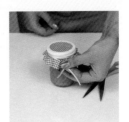

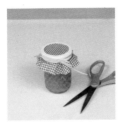

Raw jams can serve as great gift for your loved ones because they are both healthy and great tasting. They are a nice way to introduce a raw food lifestyle to other people. To package the jams nicely, follow these simple instructions:

Cut a circle out of fabric 3 inches wider than the lid of a canning jar. Place the inside of the lid on the jar. Lay the fabric circle over the inside of the lid. Screw the outer part of the lid on top of the fabric. Decorate the jar with ribbon.

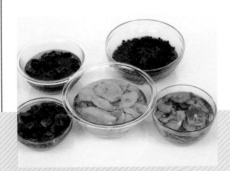

The variety of raw jams that can be prepared out of dried fruit is practically unlimited. Experiment to find your favorite!

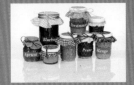

There are many ways to enjoy mango jam. Use it as you would any regular cooked jam. Raw jams on raw crackers or cookies make an excellent snack at breakfast or anytime. Served with a cup of warm herb tea, they make a cozy treat to share with a friend. Raw mango jam will keep in the refrigerator for up to two weeks. However, due to its superb taste, you will probably find it won't last that long.

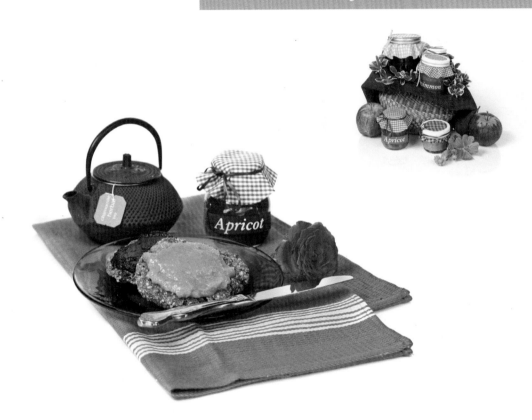

Mango jam can make a great special occasion dessert, served in fancy glasses and decorated with a slice of colorful fruit.

Raw jams have a thick consistency that also makes them perfect to use as a pie filling (see next recipe). It's handy to have some premade jam in your fridge so you can make a whole pie in minutes whenever you desire.

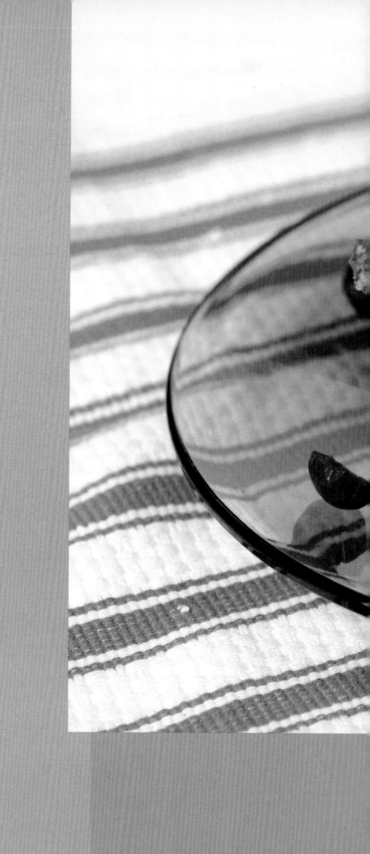

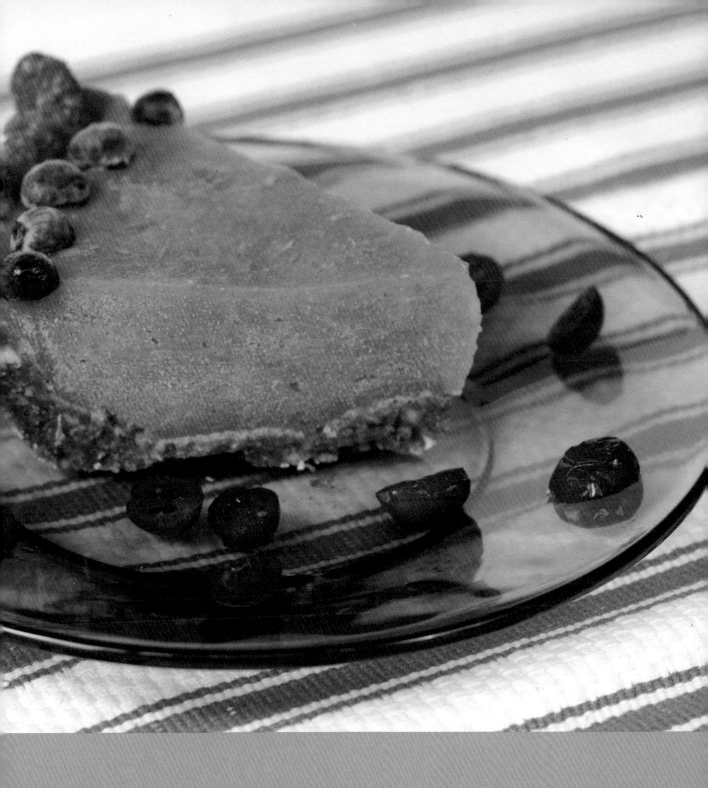

Mango Jam Pie

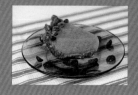

Mango Jam Pie

Jam pies are a unique Raw Family creation. These delicious pies closely resemble traditional fruit pies, the most popular American dessert.

Raw jam pies are a nutritious and guilt-free alternative to traditional fruit pies. They are sugar-free, wheat-free, dairy-free, salt-free, and oil-free! At the same time, jam pies are beautiful, delicious, and loaded with healthy nutrients. You can prepare a scrumptious mango pie with this recipe to celebrate special occasions and your health any day.

Equipment

Food processor
Bowl
Pie pan
Spatula

Ingredients

For pie crust:
3 cups almonds
1 ½ cups pitted dates
¼ cup ground nuts or dry grated coconut to sprinkle in the pie pan
For filling:
2 cups raw mango jam (see previous recipe)

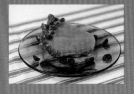

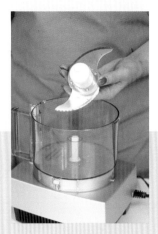

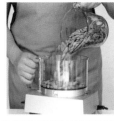

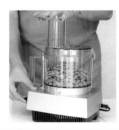

We are going to use almonds in this crust, but you may use any kind of nuts. In order to obtain the desired consistency, do not soak the nuts; rather grind them dry.

Put the S-blade into the food processor and grind the nuts to a fluffy consistency. Stop grinding when the nut powder is fine but still airy and light. With too much grinding it will become oily.

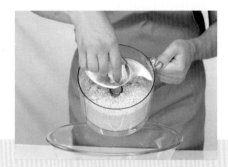

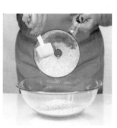

Remove the S-blade and transfer the ground nuts into a bowl using a plastic spatula or wooden spoon. (Never use metal utensils when working with your food processor. Every time you touch blades with a metal utensil, they get dulled.)

If you are using ground nuts rather than coconut to sprinkle on your pie plate, grind another ¼ cup of nuts and set them aside (see page 116).

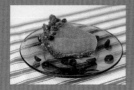

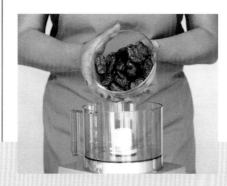

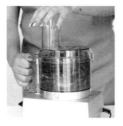

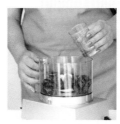

Put the dates in the food processor and grind them with the S-blade. If the dates are too dry and do not blend well, add 1 to 2 teaspoons of olive oil or lemon juice. The liquid will help the date paste blend better.

The health benefits of dates have been known since ancient times and have been recorded in the earliest scripture.

"Then he [Samuel] gave a loaf of bread, a cake of dates, and a cake of raisins to each person in the whole crowd of Israelites, both men and women." 2 Samuel 6:19 (NIV)

Muslims generally break their fast by eating dates. The prophet Muhammad is reported to have said, "If anyone of you is fasting, let him break his fast with dates. In case he does not have them, then with water."

Modern science confirms the supreme nutritional value of dates. They are rich in calcium, potassium, iron, magnesium, phosphorus, copper, manganese, and dietary fiber.

Source: www.nutritiondata.com. The information in this database comes from the USDA's National Nutrient Database for Standard Reference.

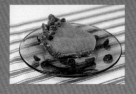

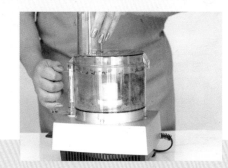
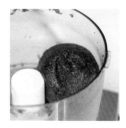
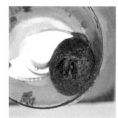
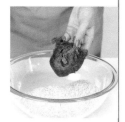

When the dates are completely blended, they will form a ball of date paste that will have a smooth consistency. Remove the date ball from the food processor and place in the bowl with the ground nuts.

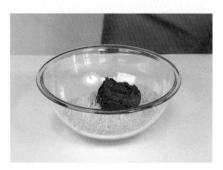
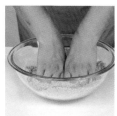
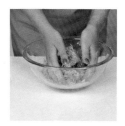
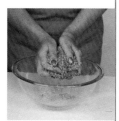

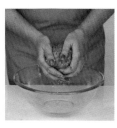
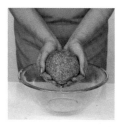

Mix the ground nuts and the date paste together with your hands. If the mixture is too dry to mix, add a little bit of water or apple juice. Don't add more than 2 to 3 tablespoons at a time. The mixture should possess an even color, be firm, fairly dry, and stick together.

115

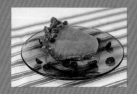

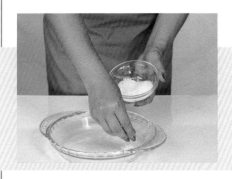

Sprinkle the shredded coconut (or ground nuts) in the pie pan. This will keep the crust from sticking to the bottom of the plate and make it much easier to serve the pie. You can also use poppy seeds, sesame seeds, buckwheat flour, or other dry coating of your choice to keep the crust from sticking to the pan.

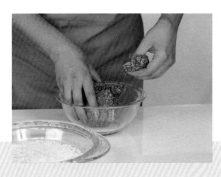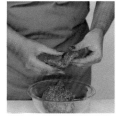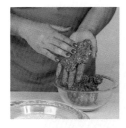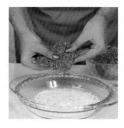

Pull off a small piece of dough and squish it into a flat patty with your palms. Make it as thin as possible. Lay the dough on top of the shredded coconut.

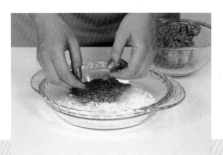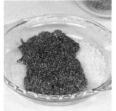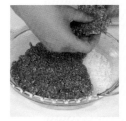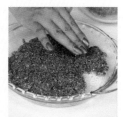

Press flat pieces of dough down to make a single, even layer. Make your pie crust as level as possible. You may find it easiest to do so by rotating the pan every once in a while to work in the place you are most comfortable.

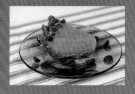

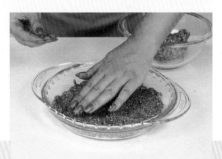

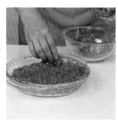

Make small patties to fill in the empty spaces as needed. Try not to miss any spaces. If you find a place where the layer is too thin, add another piece of dough.

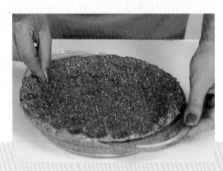

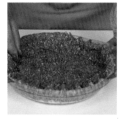

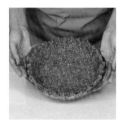

When the pie crust looks even and round, begin to create a wavy trim by pinching the edges of the crust into triangles. Make sure the triangles are touching the pie pan. This will make them stronger, and ensure that the triangles won't break off when you serve the pie. Work your way all around the pie and adjust the size of each triangle to match the others.

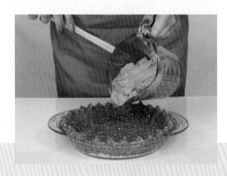

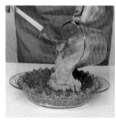

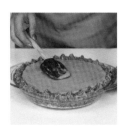

Pour your mango jam into the crust. With a spatula, spread the jam evenly over the crust, rotating the pie as needed while spreading to make the jam as level as possible. Make gentle horizontal strokes with the spatula to form a smooth, even surface. Be sure to spread the jam all the way to the edges of the pie.

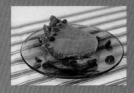
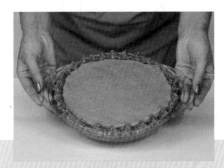
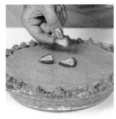
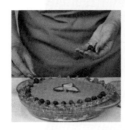
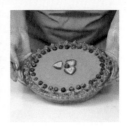

You now have a neat and traditional-looking pie. You may choose to leave your pie looking simple or to decorate it. Follow your own fancy; garnish with fresh berries, sliced fruit, or nuts.

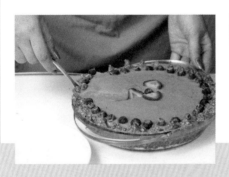
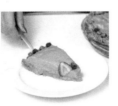

This is how beautiful a slice of your mango jam pie will look. Brightly colored, it not only looks impressive, but tastes exquisite as well.

If you would like your pie a little firmer when you serve it, place it in the refrigerator or freezer for a couple of hours. This will make the pie easier to cut, and help the slices look more defined.

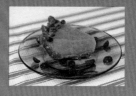

You can keep this pie in a freezer for several weeks and eat a freshly cut piece whenever you desire. A slice of mango pie is always yummy and refreshing.
Have fun!

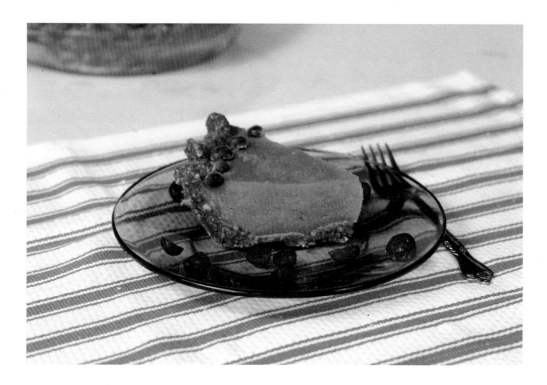

While this recipe is for mango jam pie, we invite you to play around with different variations of jam pies—blueberry, cherry, apple-cinnamon, and countless others.

A long time ago when we had just started our raw food life, we did not even know there were such things as "raw cakes." So we were thrilled when my friend Hiawatha taught us to prepare a raw dessert that she called a "peach carob cake." After practically living on salads for many months, everyone in my family savored it, despite the fact that the "cake" did not hold together and we ended up eating our liquidy slices with a spoon.

Later that day my neighbor Linda stopped by, and I offered her a "slice" of our raw peach cake. To my surprise, Linda wasn't as enthusiastic about this precious treat. I asked her, "Isn't this cake amazingly delicious?" Linda shrugged her shoulders and replied, "It's OK, but ... it is not a chocolate cake!" These words from my neighbor's lips have been echoing in my head for many years. I kept trying to create a raw cake that would be comparable to a traditional chocolate cake. In my family we came up with many different recipes for carob cakes, unchocolate cakes, and chocolate tortes. In Jamaica at a raw food showcase in 2000, we prepared a gigantic unchocolate cake that was served to two hundred guests. Gradually we acquired all the necessary tips and developed a recipe that satisfies everybody, no matter what their diet.

Today we are proud to share with you our best raw chocolate cake recipe.

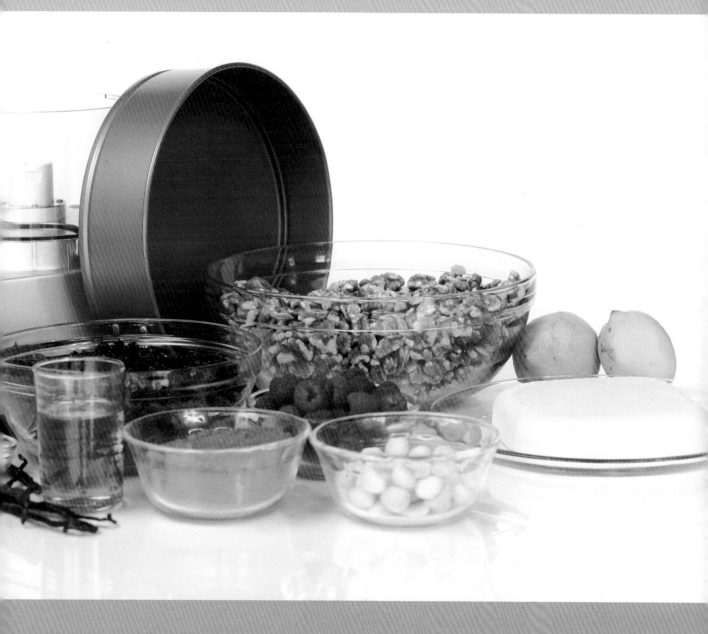

Chocolate Cake

Chocolate Cake

This chocolate cake will be the highlight of any table. Its decadent taste strikes a cord in any chocolate lover's heart. Your friends will be delighted when you serve them this mouthwatering chocolate cake.

Equipment

Food processor
Blender
Springform cake pan
Large bowl
Spatula
Cutting board
Paring knife
Plastic wrap or
    cheesecloth
Large plate

Ingredients

Ingredients for the crust:
2 cups walnuts
2 cups raisins
2 tbsp. olive oil
1 lemon
1 pint strawberries
2 pears
Ingredients for the frosting:
1 lemon
1 cup pecans
½ cup raw agave nectar
¼ tsp. sea salt (optional)
4 tbsp. raw cacao powder
1 vanilla bean
1 handful of shredded coconut

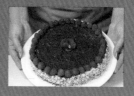

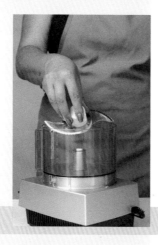

Place the S-shaped blade in the food processor.

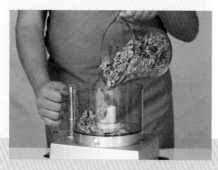

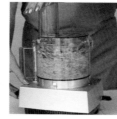

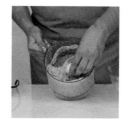

Pour the walnuts into the food processor, secure the lid, and grind the nuts to a powder.

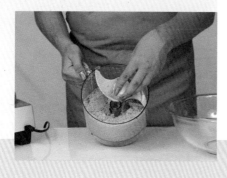

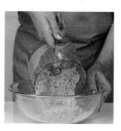

Remove the blade and pour the ground walnuts into a large bowl.

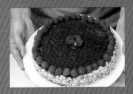

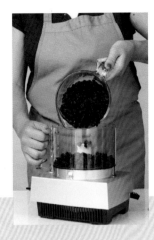 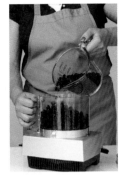 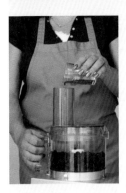

Put the S-blade back into the food processor, add the raisins, and pour in the olive oil.

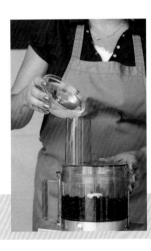

Juice one lemon and pour the juice into the food processor. Blend well until the consistency is creamy.

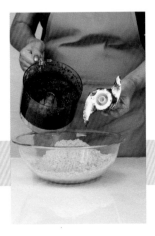 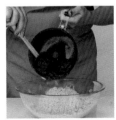 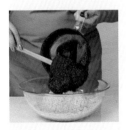

Remove the blade and use a spatula to scrape out the batter and add it to the ground walnuts.

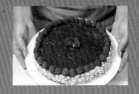
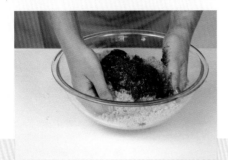

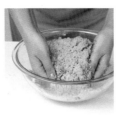

Using both hands, knead the ingredients together into dough. Pray, meditate, think positive thoughts, or sing while kneading your dough!

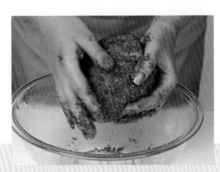

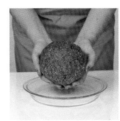

You will end up with a nice firm ball of perfectly mixed dough for the cake.

Divide your cake dough into three equal parts, one for each layer.

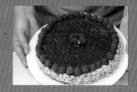

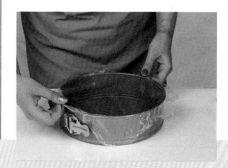 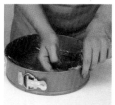

Position plastic wrap or cheesecloth inside the Springform pan.

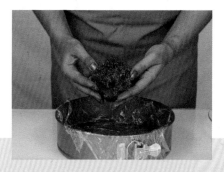 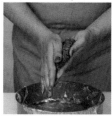 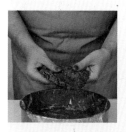 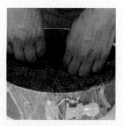

Break off a chunk of dough, flatten it between your palms, and press it into the cake pan with your hands. Keep adding more flattened pieces of dough until the entire bottom is covered with a thin layer of cake dough.

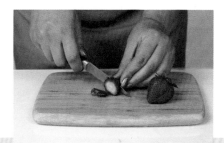 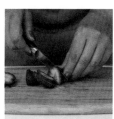 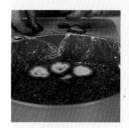 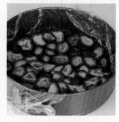

Slice the strawberries and arrange them on top of the dough layer. Place the strawberries as closely together as you can, covering as much of the surface as possible.

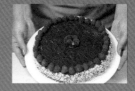

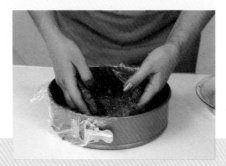

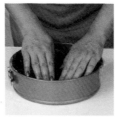

For the second layer, break pieces from your second portion of cake dough. Flatten the pieces between your palms and lightly place them on top of the strawberries. Do not push them down; you don't want to squeeze juice out of the strawberries.

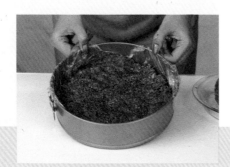

When all the strawberries are covered with a dough layer without any holes, you are ready for the next layer of fruit.

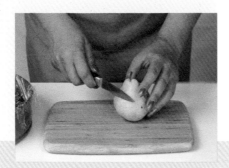

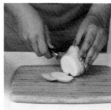

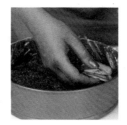

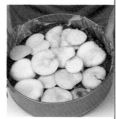

Cut the pears into thin flat slices and arrange them on top of the second layer of dough.

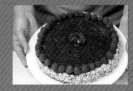

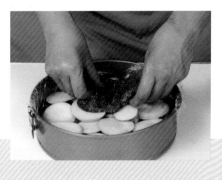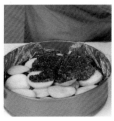

Use the third portion of dough to form a final layer on top of the pears. Make sure the whole cake is covered with dough.

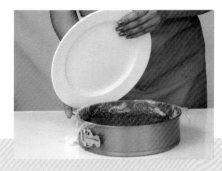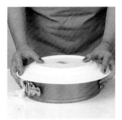

Position the large plate over the pan as shown in the picture. With both your hands, firmly hold the pan and plate together and quickly turn them over. Open the Springform pan. Your cake will drop down about an inch.

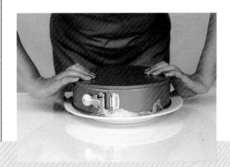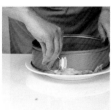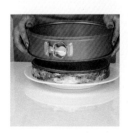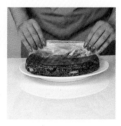

Carefully lift off the outer ring and gently peel the plastic wrap or cheesecloth off the cake.

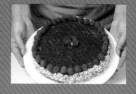

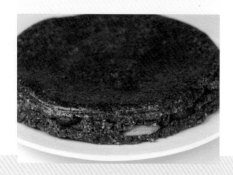

This is our basic cake. Now we need to make chocolate frosting.

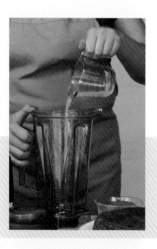

The easiest way to make the frosting is in a high-speed blender as shown in these pictures. If you have a regular blender, you might need to grind the nuts separately in a coffee grinder prior to blending.

Pour the juice of one lemon into the blender.

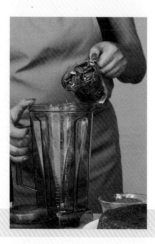

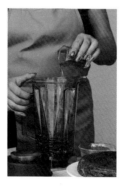

Add the pecans and the raw agave nectar.

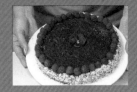
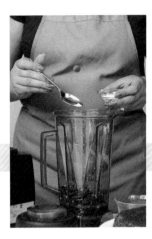 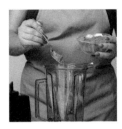 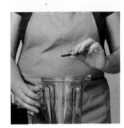

Add the salt, raw cacao powder, and vanilla bean.

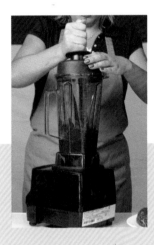 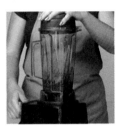

Secure the lid and blend well. If you have a tamper (often sold together with blenders), you will find it helpful in processing this thick-consistency frosting.

  If your mixture is too dry to blend, add water or lemon juice slowly in very small amounts, using a teaspoon. If the frosting is too liquidy, it won't stay on the sides of the cake.

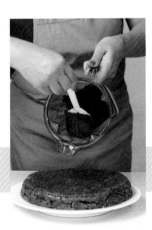 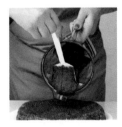 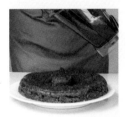

With a spatula, scoop your chocolate frosting onto the cake.

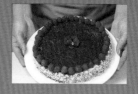

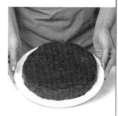

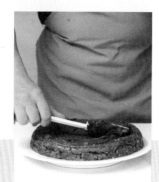

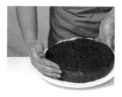

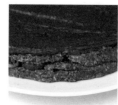

Spread the frosting evenly over the top of the cake and then work your way around the sides.

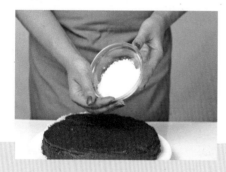

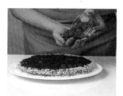

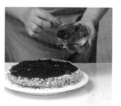

To give the cake a professionally made look, we like to cover the sides of the cake with ground coconut. Take a handful of coconut shreds and sprinkle it evenly on the sides of the cake, rotating the plate with your other hand as you go.

Decorate as you desire with fresh fruits, berries, or edible flowers.

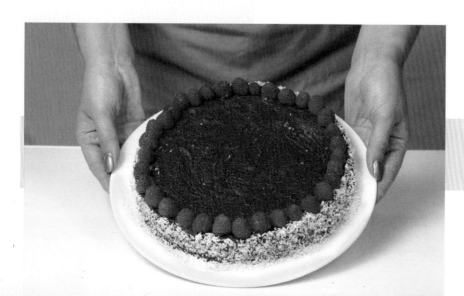

Chill the cake in the refrigerator for a few hours for easy slicing.

131

The traditional (cooked) mousse cake is a favorite treat for many dessert lovers. However, not many people are aware that one slice (218 g, or 7.7 ounces) of a typical chocolate mousse cake contains on average 1,950 calories.[1] According to scientific research, 3,500 calories equals one pound of fat.[2] That means a slice and a half of that mousse cake can add a pound of fat to one's hips. Remember, it's much faster to gain that weight than to lose it again!

The good news is that the following raw mousse cake recipe contains six times fewer calories than a typical mousse cake. One slice of our cake contains about 322 calories but is still highly competitive with a traditional mousse cake both in taste and appearance. Moreover, this cake is wheat-free, sugar-free, egg-free, dairy-free, and is loaded with healthy, raw nutrients.

Even so, I would like to clarify that cake, even if it is a raw creation, cannot substitute nutritionally for green smoothies and salads. We believe that all desserts have to be eaten sparingly. But on special occasions you will greatly enjoy these tasty raw concoctions.

1. www.nutritiondata.com
2. www.health.gov/dietaryguidelines

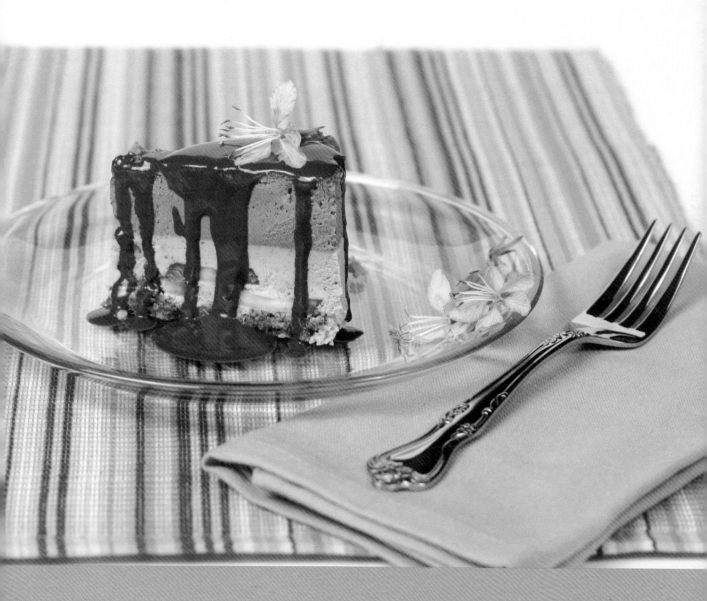

Mousse Cake

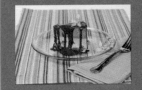

Mousse Cake

We now offer you our perfected-over-the-years recipe of a mousse cake that you can rely on for any holiday. You don't even have to mention that your cake is raw; your loved ones will not be disappointed. We shared our raw mousse cake with lots of our friends and everyone loved it. Please follow the directions carefully and enjoy!

Equipment

Food processor
Blender
Springform cake pan
Large bowl
Spatula
Cutting board
Paring knife
Large plate

Ingredients

2 cups water
1 cup dough for the cake (see Chocolate Cake recipe, page 121)
3 tbsp. shredded coconut or powdered nuts
1 cup strawberries
½ cup macadamia nuts or cashews
1 cup cacao butter or coconut butter
1 cup raw agave nectar
½ cup cranberries or raspberries (fresh or frozen)
1 vanilla bean
1 small piece of raw beet, approximately 1 x ½ inches
¼ tsp. sea salt (optional)
4 tbsp. raw cacao powder

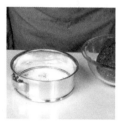

Prepare the dough for your mousse cake by following the directions on page 122. You will need only half of the dough from the chocolate cake recipe, so cut all of those ingredients in half, or else make two mousse cakes, or use the extra dough to make truffles.

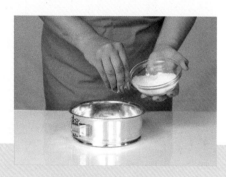

Sprinkle shredded coconut or ground nuts on the bottom of a Springform cake pan so the cake won't stick to it.

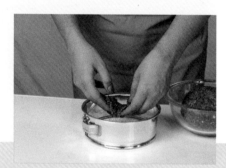

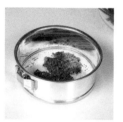

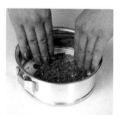

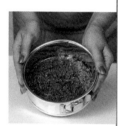

Break off a chunk of dough and flatten it between your palms. Lay thin pieces of dough into the cake pan. Keep adding more flattened chunks of dough until the entire bottom is covered with a thin layer of cake dough.

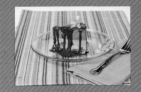

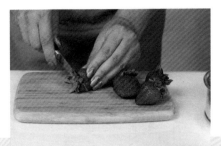 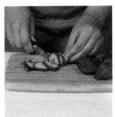 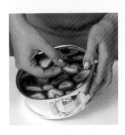 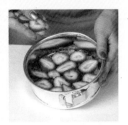

Slice the strawberries and arrange the slices on top of the dough layer. Place the strawberries as closely together as you can, covering as much of the surface as possible.

Now let's prepare two different kinds of mousse—cranberry and chocolate—to make our cake delicious and beautiful.

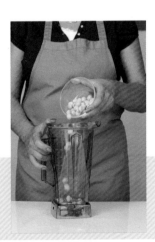 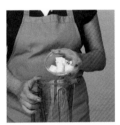

To make the cranberry mousse, first grind the macadamia nuts. If you have a regular blender, you might need to grind the nuts separately in a coffee grinder prior to blending them with the other ingredients.

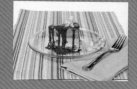

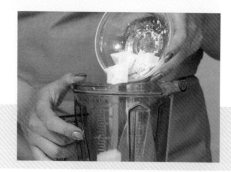

Put half of the cacao butter or coconut butter into your blender. Make sure that your butter is broken into chunks no bigger than 1 inch in size.

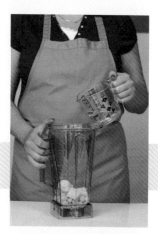

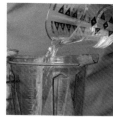

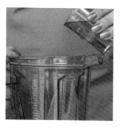

Pour in 1 cup of water and ½ cup raw agave nectar. (You will use the rest in the next layer.)

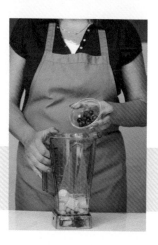

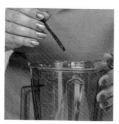

Add the cranberries and half of the vanilla bean. If you cannot get a vanilla bean, you may use 1 tsp. vanilla extract.

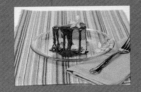
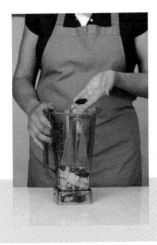

Cut a very small slice of red beet (peeled), approximately 1 inch long and ½ inch thick. Red beet will tint your mousse a beautiful light pink color.

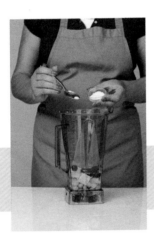
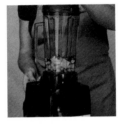
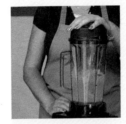

Add salt, then secure the lid and blend well for at least 1 minute, or until all the chunks of butter are completely whipped.

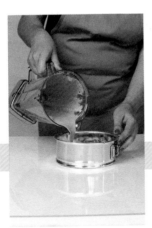
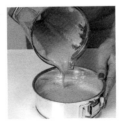

Pour your mousse on top of the strawberry layer.

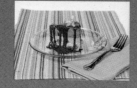

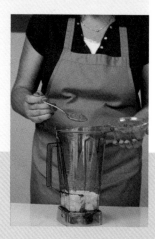

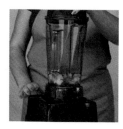

To prepare the chocolate mousse, put the remaining cacao butter or coconut butter into your blender. (Make sure that your butter is broken into chunks no bigger than 1 inch in size.)

Add 1 cup of water, ½ cup agave nectar, the cacao powder, and the other half of the vanilla bean (or 1 tsp. vanilla extract). Secure the lid and blend well for at least 1 minute, or until all the chunks of butter are completely whipped.

If your kitchen is very warm, you may want to place your cake in the freezer for a few minutes to solidify before pouring the next mousse layer.

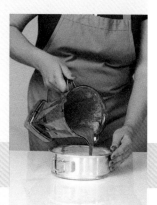

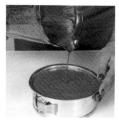

Pour your chocolate mousse on top of the pink mousse layer.

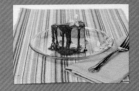

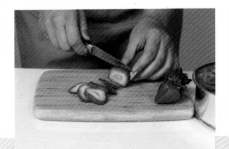
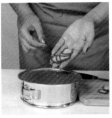
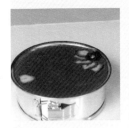
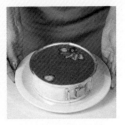

Decorate the cake with strawberry slices and an edible flower.

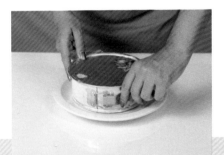
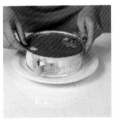
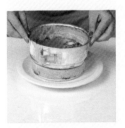
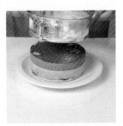

With the large plate and cake positioned as shown in the picture, open the Springform pan and carefully lift off the outer ring.

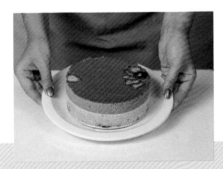
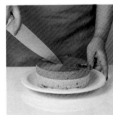
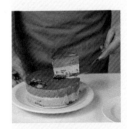

You may want to chill your cake before serving for easier slicing.

If you would like to make a chocolate sauce to drizzle on your mousse cake, blend 1 teaspoon of raw cacao powder with ¼ cup agave nectar. Use a tablespoon for drizzling onto cut slices.

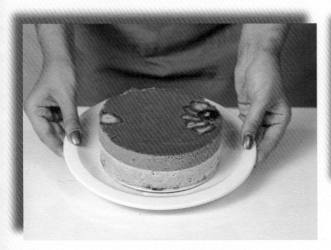
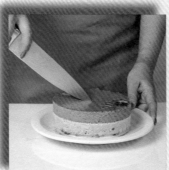
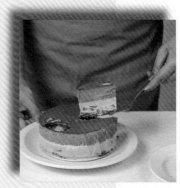
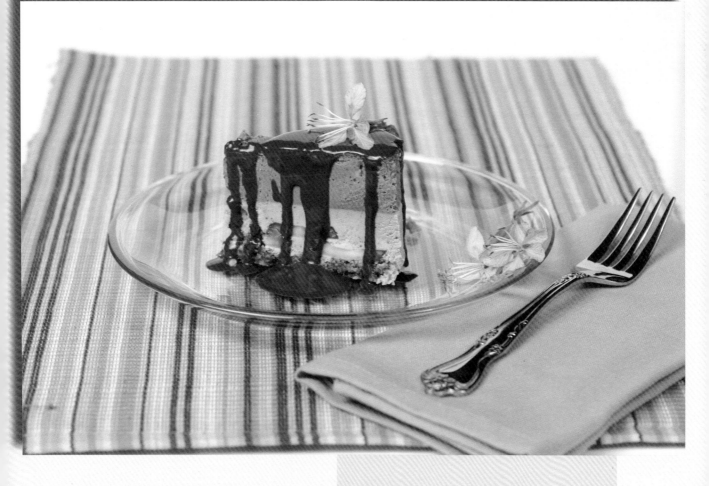

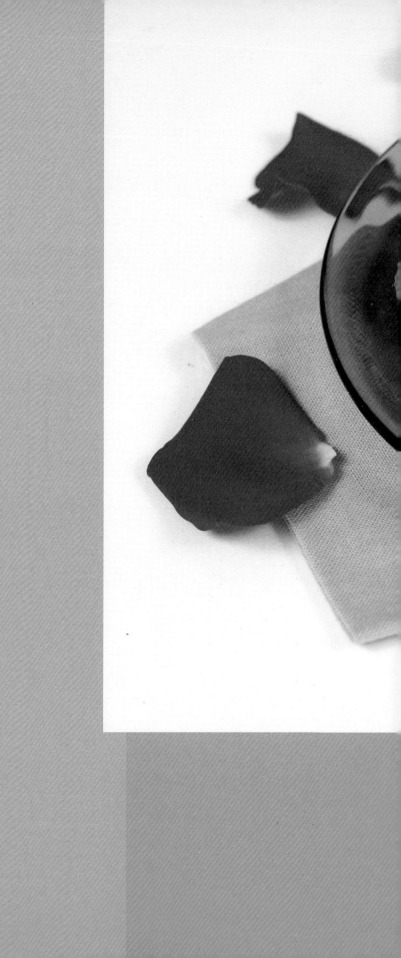

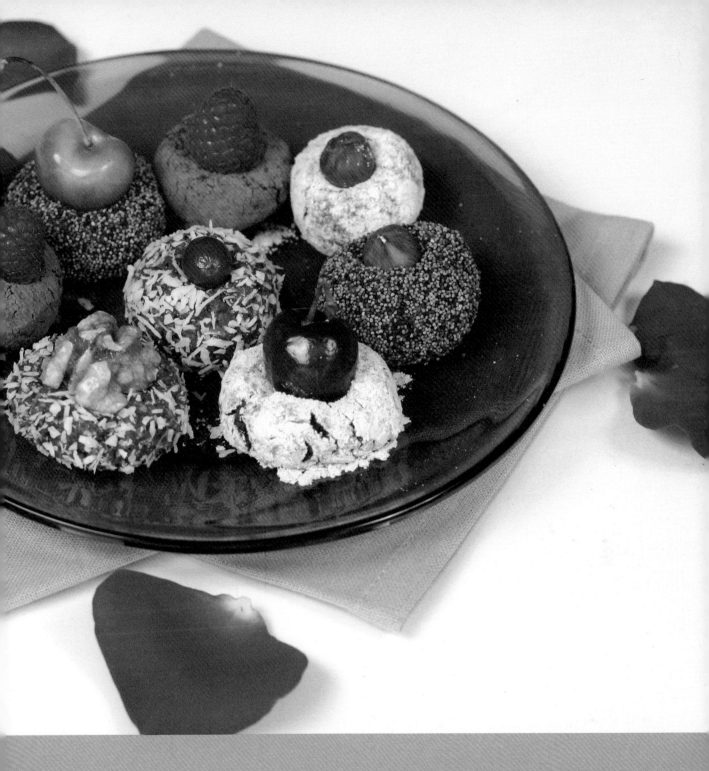

Chocolate Truffles

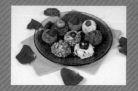
Chocolate Truffles

This decadent dessert is attractive and delicious, yet healthy and simple to make. Presented in a box with a bow, these truffles make a memorable gift.

Equipment

Coffee grinder
Five small bowls
Serving plate

Ingredients

2 tbsp. raw sesame seeds (hulled or unhulled)
2 tbsp. poppy seeds
2 tbsp. shredded coconut
2 tbsp. raw cacao or carob powder
2 tbsp. raw oat flour (grind rolled oats in coffee grinder)
2 cups chocolate cake dough (see page 122)
Assortment of nuts and berries for decoration

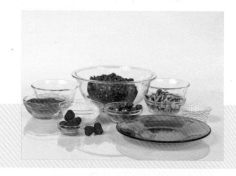

Pour the sesame seeds, poppy seeds, shredded coconut, cacao powder, and oat flour into separate small bowls. These will be the coatings for your truffles.

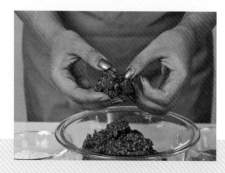

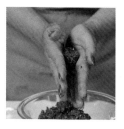

Pinch off a piece of cake dough approximately 1 inch in diameter and roll it into a smooth ball.

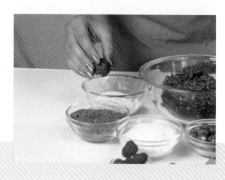

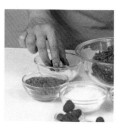

Dip the ball into one of the coatings, rolling until it is evenly coated.

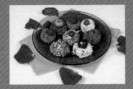
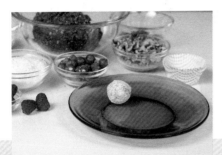 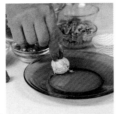 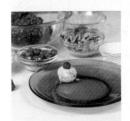

Place the coated ball on a plate and press a nut of your choice into the coated ball.

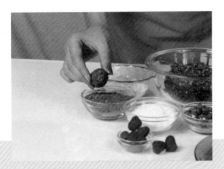 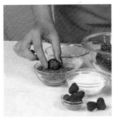 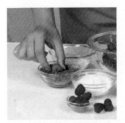 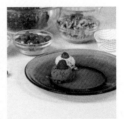

Pinch off another piece of cake dough approximately 1 inch in diameter and roll it in a different coating.

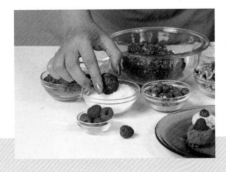 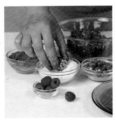

Keep making balls of the same size and rolling them in the different coatings until the dough is used up.

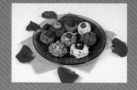

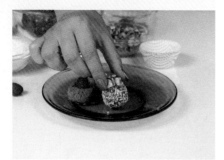
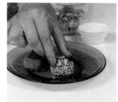
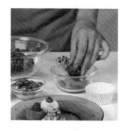
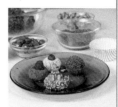
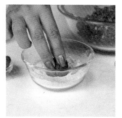
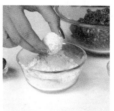

If you are going to decorate your truffle with a raspberry or other soft fruit, first make an indentation with your finger before placing the fruit.

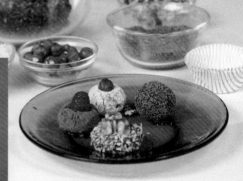

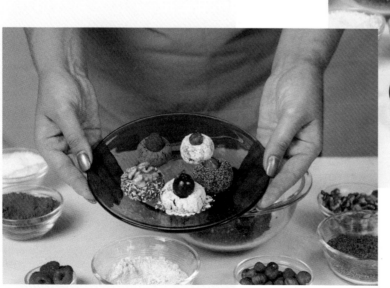

Decorate the plate with flower petals before serving.

Makes approximately 12 truffles.

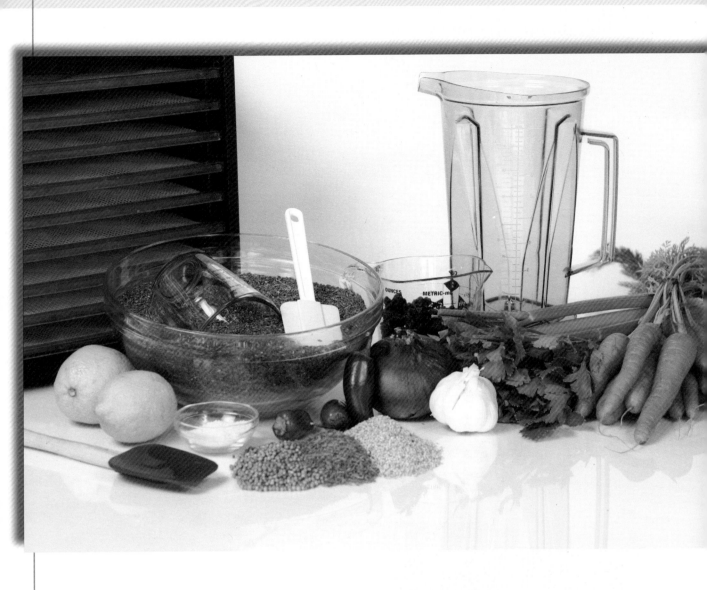

Equipment List

[adapted from *Fresh: The Ultimate Live-Food Cookbook,* with permission from Sergei and Valya Boutenko]

Every ordinary kitchen contains the necessary tools for food preparation. A raw food kitchen is no different. However, instead of a stove, pots, pans, eggbeaters, and oven mitts, a raw food kitchen relies on a cutting board, a good set of knives, a blender, a food processor, and a dehydrator. This section is dedicated to the equipment that makes up a traditional raw food kitchen. While having the following equipment will make your transition to a plant-based diet easier, more enjoyable, and less stressful, it is by no means essential. Like a new kitchen stove, a superior quality blender often comes with a high price tag, which is unrealistic for many people. If your household is low on funds, rest assured that you can make do with whatever equipment you can get your hands on. For example, if you own a blender that is not as powerful as a Vita-Mix, that's OK! Simply blend your concoction longer, until it reaches a satisfying consistency. Ultimately the decision is yours, and whatever you decide is right.

With the huge variety of blenders, food processors, and dehydrators on the market today, it can seem impossible to know which are the best to purchase. With prices ranging from fifteen to seven hundred dollars, how can you be certain that choosing one brand over another ensures a quality product at a reasonable price? We have tested all the appliances mentioned below over the course of fifteen years in hundreds of food preparation demonstrations. Having created literally thousands of recipes using various machines, we weeded out each piece of equipment that was less than perfect until left with the absolute best. All of the items discussed below are tools that we use and recommend.

Vita-Mix Blender $249–599

A blender is used for completely crushing up and liquefying ingredients to create dishes such as smoothies, soups, dressings, sauces, pie toppings, and puddings. Because many raw ingredients are rich in fiber and cellulose (a very tough plant matter), liquefying them often requires high levels of power and strength. We wholeheartedly recommend buying a Vita-Mix blender, because it meets our requirement for strength and power better than any other mixer on the market. While common blenders mix at roughly 11 miles per hour, the Vita-Mix rotates at 240 miles per hour. Essentially, this means that if you dump some wooden blocks into a Vita-Mix container and add water, you will have a creamy log soup.

In a more practical application, the Vita-Mix blender allows you to play around with consistency, resulting in everything from a chunky mixture (often preferred for soups) to a fluffy, creamy mixture (great for sweets, cake frosting, and puddings). Furthermore, the Vita-Mix can replace the need for a juicer when the liquefied matter is strained through a strainer or nut-milk bag, separating the liquid from the solid.

If you place dried nuts, seeds, or grains into a Vita-Mix and blend them without water, the machine will pulverize these ingredients into flour. This is extremely handy for making garden burgers, pâté, hummus, and crackers. All around, the Vita-Mix is the most versatile piece of equipment, so if you can only afford one appliance, we advise you to start with the Vita-Mix blender.

Vita-Mix Resources

Vita-Mix	www.rawfamily.com	1-800-848-2649

Epinions   www.epinions.com
A convenient Web site for comparing kitchen appliances

Cuisinart Food Processor $100–200

Like a blender, a food processor grinds ingredients into smaller pieces. However, while a blender liquefies all ingredients, a food processor chops food into smaller pieces. With a wider holding container and S-shaped blades that don't extend to the edges of the container, the food processor becomes the perfect tool for making such foods as pâté, hummus, guacamole, pie crusts, and burgers. Food processors usually come with several handy additional blades, including a grater and a slicer, which are perfect for making specialty salads, chips, and marinated foods.

We recommend buying a Cuisinart over other brands because not only are Cuisinarts strong and durable, their blades are made from higher-quality metal that stays sharp longer. These blades easily grind through hard vegetables, nuts, seeds, and grains.

There are several different models available. We recommend the simple seven-cup model because we find it to be the most efficient and user-friendly. This model costs less and does not include a glut of puzzle pieces needing to be assembled for the machine to function properly.

Cuisinart Resources

Cuisinart	www.cuisinart.com	1-800-726-0190
Everything Kitchens	www.everythingkitchens.com	1-866-852-4268
Amazon.com	www.amazon.com	
Epinions	www.epinions.com	

A convenient Web site for comparing kitchen appliances

Excalibur Dehydrator $109–250

A dehydrator can be considered the oven of the raw food kitchen, except instead of using extreme heat to process food, a dehydrator, or dryer, blows warm air (usually around body temperature, 98 degrees F) over food in a contained environment. This process draws water out of food, thereby preserving it and concentrating its flavor.

Food dryers are essential for making such snacks as chips, crackers, breads, cookies, and travel foods. If you like dried fruit or happen to obtain an abundance of overripe produce, you can create delicious, nutrient-rich snacks by dehydrating them.

Of all the dehydrators we have tested, our favorite is the Excalibur. Not only is it reasonably priced for a commercial dehydrator, but it is also made with exceptional craftsmanship and ingenuity. Unlike its competition, the Excalibur is built with the heating fan placed vertically and at the back of the unit, which ensures that every tray receives an even amount of heat regardless of whether it is located at the top, middle, or bottom. The end product is consistently dried, tasty food.

One of the best features of the Excalibur is that its temperature can be adjusted by a dial on top of the unit. While the basic rule of thumb is to try to dry everything as close to body temperature as possible, one should be aware of several exceptions. For example, when drying moisture-rich foods such as melons and tomatoes, cranking the heat up to 112–115 degrees F for the first six hours prevents these foods from getting moldy. The presence of moisture in the food keeps its inside temperature lower than that of the air in the dehydrator.

Finally, it is important to note that Excalibur has several different models on the market. We recommend the nine-tray model, the 2900. There are smaller, cheaper models; however, they all draw approximately the same amount of electricity as this one and don't cost significantly less. With the nine-tray model, you can make food in large batches, preventing the need to make a mess in your kitchen every other day. In the long run, even if you live alone, having nine trays is much more practical.

Excalibur Dehydrator Resources

Excalibur	www.excaliburdehydrator.com	1-800-875-4254
Canning Pantry	www.canningpantry.com	1-800-285-9044
Kitchen Universe	www.kitchen-universe.com	1-877-517-1966
Become	www.become.com	

Another convenient Web site for comparing kitchen appliances

Champion Juicer $180–259

A juicer extracts liquids from fruits and vegetables, and separates the pulp. Juicers are not generally considered versatile machines because most are engineered for the sole task of extracting juice. This is starting to change as more and more companies start designing juicers for various other tasks.

The Champion juicer is our favorite because it includes several attachments that allow you to make ice cream, nut butters, and pâtés in addition to juices. Juicers tend to be complicated, with lots of little pieces needing to be assembled prior to using them, but the Champion juicer has a total of five pieces that are easy to assemble and clean.

Champion Juicer Resources

Champion Juicer	www.championjuicer.com	1-866-935-8423
On the World Wide Web	www.discountjuicers.com	
HealthWisdom	www.healthwisdom.com	1-888-337-8646
Rhio's Raw Energy	www.rawfoodinfo.com	1-212-941-5857

Veggie Spiralizer $25–100

A spiralizer is used to shred vegetables and hard fruits into noodle form. This tool makes it easy to create dishes such as lasagna, pasta, and macaroni. Unlike a regular grater, a veggie spiralizer has different blades that help process food into beautiful, symmetrical shapes and sizes. Furthermore, spiralizers have a built-in mechanism that prevents veggies from ripping, ensuring a long and continuous noodle strand. Of the numerous spiralizer models available, we have used many different ones and liked them all.

Veggie Spiralizer Resources

Livingnutrition	www.livingnutrition.com	1-707-829-0462
Raw Life	www.rawlife.com	1-866-Raw-Paul (729-7285)
Target	www.target.com	
NaturalZing	www.naturalzing.com	1-301-703-4116

Nut-Milk Bag $8–12

Nut-milk bags are used to strain liquid away from fibrous, pulpy material. A nut-milk bag is a wonderful tool that each household should have on hand. This simple device can ease the process of making nut and seed milks, juices, pâtés, cookies, and sprouts. There are many online sources that sell nut-milk bags; however, it is extremely easy to make one, so it's a good idea to consider this option before buying.

To make a nut-milk bag, you need to obtain some sort of mesh or loose-knit natural fiber and a drawstring, and have access to a sewing machine. By folding the mesh into a square, sewing around the edges, and adding a drawstring to the top, you can create a cheap and efficient nut-milk bag and begin straining away!

Nut-Milk Bag Resources

Raw Family	www.rawfamily.com	1-541-488-8865

Cutting Board $1–40

A cutting board does not require much explanation; it is a board for cutting food! Since raw food requires quite a lot of cutting, we recommend finding a cutting board that works for you and your living situation. This may be a thick wooden cutting board or a thin malleable one. There is no right or wrong, so choose freely. The bottom line is that you and the board will develop a relationship in the coming years. To help you follow through on your commitment to raw foods, you may want to find a board that you love from the very beginning!

Cutting Board Resources

Amazon.com   www.amazon.com

Ross Dress for Less   www.rossstores.com
Carries a variety of high-quality, low-priced cutting boards

Chef's Resource   www.chefsresource.com   1-866-765-Chef (2433)

The Cutting Board Company
                         www.cuttingboardcompany.com   1-866-247-2409

Knives $2–200

As mentioned previously, raw food requires massive amounts of cutting. Find a knife or set of knives that you like and keep them in a convenient place. The price of a set of knives does not necessarily indicate good quality or whether you will like them. We have used hundreds of knives in various price ranges and have come to the conclusion that buying cheap knives is a waste of money because they get dull fast, leech unhealthy materials into food, and can be potentially dangerous to work with.

On the other hand, purchasing expensive knives may cause you unnecessary worry that something might happen to them. The best knives that have graced our hands have always been within the fifteen-to-twenty-dollar range. They are sharp and have a comfortable handle and a reasonable weight (not too heavy or light), which is what we look for when knife shopping. But you should shop around to discover your favorite kind; people often have very strong preferences about what works for them. Stores like Sur La Table or Williams-Sonoma usually have a big selection of knives that you can

get the feel of in your hand. Certainly you don't need to decide on a whole collection!
One or two good knives will do the trick for most of your needs.

Knife Resources

Amazon.com   www.amazon.com

Index

Acknowledgments

I would like to acknowledge my beloved family for their contribution of recipes to this book. Thank you for always being there for me.

I sincerely appreciate the skill and dedication of Robert Petetit, master photographer and friend, and his hundreds of hours of work shooting and editing the pictures in this book.

I'm grateful to Alison's of Ashland for lending me their lovely dishes.

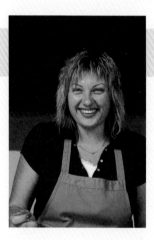

A special thank you goes out to my sister Marina for being a perfect model, for her patience, hard work, and beautiful hands.

About the Author

Victoria Boutenko lives in Ashland, Oregon. She is the award-winning author of *Green For Life, Raw Family,* and *12 Steps to Raw Foods.* Victoria is a raw gourmet chef, teacher, inventor, researcher, and artist. She teaches classes on healthy living all over the world. As a result of her teachings, millions of people are drinking green smoothies and eating raw food internationally. She continues traveling worldwide sharing her gourmet raw cuisine and her inspiring story of determination. To learn more about Victoria and raw foods, please visit www.rawfamily.com.